499 Powerful Hypnotic Affirmations and Spiritual Self-Care for Black Women:

2 in 1 Book: Feminine Daily Affirmations for Motivation, Confidence, Positivity, and Money. Overcome Anxiety and Depression

Feminine Positive Affirmations for Black Women:

Become Divine Women and Live a Life in Abundance and Joy. Increase Self-Love, Wealth, Success and Self-Esteem Forever.

© Copyright 2022 by CHASECHECK LTD - All rights reserved.

The content contained within this book may not be reproduced, duplicated or transmitted without direct written permission from the author or the publisher.

Under no circumstances will any blame or legal responsibility be held against the publisher, or author, for any damages, reparation, or monetary loss due to the information contained within this book. Either directly or indirectly.

Legal Notice:

This book is copyright protected. This book is only for personal use. You cannot amend, distribute, sell, use, quote or paraphrase any part, or the content within this book, without the consent of the author or publisher.

Disclaimer Notice:

Please note the information contained within this document is for educational and entertainment purposes only. All effort has been executed to present accurate, up to date, and reliable, complete information. No warranties of any kind are declared or implied. Readers acknowledge that the author is not engaging in the rendering of legal, financial, medical or professional advice. The content within this book has been derived from various sources. Please consult a licensed professional before attempting any techniques outlined in this book.

By reading this document, the reader agrees that under no circumstances is the author responsible for any losses, direct or indirect, which are incurred as a result of the use of information contained within this document, including, but not limited to, — errors, omissions, or inaccuracies.

Contents

INTRODUCTION

CHAPTER ONE ix

    Beyond The Surface ix

    RELIGION AND SPIRITUALITY 4

    EMOTIONAL HEALTH AND SPIRITUALITY xv

    IMPACTS OF SPIRITUALITY ON MENTAL HEALTH xvi

    IMPROVING SPIRITUAL HEALTH xviii

    AFFIRMATIONS FOR SPIRITUALITY xix

    KEY POINTS xx

CHAPTER TWO xxii

    SELF AWARENESS xxii

    WHY DO I NEED TO KNOW MYSELF? xxiv

    Self-Love xxv

    Independence xxvi

    Clear Decision Making xxvi

    LEARNING ABOUT YOURSELF xxviii

    Be Still xxix

    Distinguish Between Who You Are And Who You Want To Be xxix

    Find Out Your Strengths And Weaknesses xxx

    Follow Your Passion xxxi

    AFFIRMATIONS FOR SELF AWARENESS xxxi

    KEY POINTS xxxiii

CHAPTER THREE xxxiv

    SEXUALITY xxxiv

    Female Sexual Problems xxxvi

    Causes Of Female Sexual Problems xxxvii

Diagnosis Of Female Sexual Problems xxxviii

Prevention Of Female Sexual Problems xl

LIVING ABOVE THE STIGMA OF STDS xli

Honesty Is Key xli

Importance of Breaking The Stigma xliii

Affirmations For A Positive Sexual Health xliv

Key Points xlv

CHAPTER FOUR .... **xlvii**

WORKPLACE xlvii

Home Office xlviii

Farm or Outdoor Location xlix

Store xlix

PURPOSE OF THE WORKPLACE xlix

WORKPLACE STRUGGLES li

Sexual Harassment lii

Kiss up, Kick down liii

Gender Inequality liv

The Toxic Workplace lv

Fatigue and Ill Health lvi

Lack of Enthusiasm lvii

Low Turnover Rate lvii

Stifled Growth lvii

COPING WITH WORKPLACE TOXICITY lvii

Find Support lvii

Stay Positive lviii

Take a Break lix

Meditate lix

Surround Yourself With Positivity lix
Quit lix
AFFIRMATIONS lx
KEY POINTS... lxi

CHAPTER FIVE .... **lxii**
FRIENDSHIPS lxii
WHAT ARE FRIENDSHIPS?.......................................lxiii
FORMS OF FRIENDSHIPS lxiv
So What Does He Say? lxv
Friendships Of Utility.. lxv
Friendship of Pleasure... lxvii
Friendships Of The Good lxviii
QUALITIES OF A FRIEND lxx
Loyalty lxx
Trust Worthiness.. lxxi
Acceptance.. lxxi
Listening Ears... lxxii
Reciprocity.. lxxii
AFFIRMATIONS lxxiv
KEY POINTS.. lxxv

CHAPTER SIX lxxv
FINANCES.. lxxv
PERSONAL FINANCES lxxvii
Essence of Personal Finances.......................................lxxvii
Meeting Money Needs... lxxix
Managing Your Income lxxix
Budgeting, Spending, Saving, and Investing lxxx

Having the Family Financially Secured lxxxi
Keeping Off Bad Debts lxxxii
Improving the Standard of Living lxxxii
RULES OF PERSONAL FINANCE lxxxiii
Have a Goal lxxxiii
Start Saving Early lxxxiii
Distinguish Wants From Needs lxxxiv
Differentiate between Assets and Liabilities lxxxiv
Live Within Your Means lxxxiv
Don't Invest in Anything You Don't Understand lxxxv
Settle Debts With the Highest Interest Rate First lxxxv
Prepare for Emergencies lxxxv
Educate Yourself lxxxvi
AFFIRMATIONS lxxxvii
CHAPTER SEVEN lxxxix
THE CAREER WOMAN lxxxix
A JOB AND A CAREER xci
Requirements xciii
Time xciii
Income xcv
CAREER DEVELOPMENT xcv
THE STAGES OF CAREER DEVELOPMENT xcv
Self-Assessment xcvi
Career Awareness xcvi
Goal-Setting xcvi
Skill Training xcvii
Performing xcvii

FACTORS INFLUENCING CAREER DEVELOPMENT.........xcvii
Personal Characteristics.. xcviii
Physical and Mental Abilities..................................... xcviii
Socio-Economic Factors.. xcix
Chance Factors xcix
IMPROVING YOUR CAREER DEVELOPMENT xcix
Learn Everyday c
Be Indispensable c
Interaction c
Figure out your Weaknesses ci
Be Yourself, Always ci
POSITIVE CAREER AFFIRMATIONS ci
KEY POINTS ciii

CHAPTER EIGHT civ
THE WOMAN LEADER.. civ
WHO IS A LEADER?... cv
QUALITIES OF A LEADER cv
A Sense of Purpose cv
Empathy cvi
Vision cvi
Creativity cvii
Motivation cvii
Making Room for Improvement cviii
Communication cviii
LEADERSHIP MISCONCEPTIONS cix
WOMEN IN LEADERSHIP... cx
Value for Balance cxi

They are More Empathetic cxi
Great Multitaskers cxii
Better Communicators cxii
Flexibility cxii
Inclusiveness cxiii
Emotional Intelligence cxiii
Ability to Handle Crises... cxiv
Defying the Odds cxiv
POSITIVE AFFIRMATIONS FOR LEADERSHIP cxv
KEY POINTS... cxvi
CHAPTER NINE............. Error! Bookmark not defined.
THE BLACK WOMAN AND BEAUTY cxvii
BEAUTY.. cxviii
    General Overview of Beauty cxviii
BEAUTY; THE INSECURITY..................................... cxix
Low Self-Esteem cxx
Overthinking... cxxi
Self-Condemnation.. cxxii
Self-Isolation cxxii
Desperation cxxiii
Exercise Daily cxxiv
Skin and Haircare, Manicure, and Pedicure............. cxxiv
Go Shopping cxxv
Keep Records cxxv
Share with Others.. cxxvi
Black Beauty cxxvi
POSITIVE AFFIRMATIONS FOR BEAUTY cxxix

KEY POINTS...cxxx

CHAPTER TEN cxxxi

A HEALTHY MIND... cxxxi

THE MIND IS DISSECTED cxxxii

TAKING CONTROL cxxxvii

Acceptance... cxxxviii

Switch POVs cxxxix

Positivity Always! cxl

POSITIVE AFFIRMATIONS FOR A HEALTHY MIND cxli

KEY POINTS.. cxliii

CHAPTER ELEVEN cxliv

BLACK WOMEN ENTREPRENEURS........................ cxliv

WHO IS AN ENTREPRENEUR? cxliv

GISELLE KNOWLES-CARTER cxlv

LYNDA RAE RESNICK cxlvi

OPRAH WINFREY cxlvii

MADAME C.J WALKER cxlvii

DANA ELAINE OWENS cxlviii

SMALL BUSINESSES..cxlix

SCALABLE STARTUPS cxlix

SOCIAL ENTREPRENEURSHIP cl

WHAT DOES IT TAKE TO BE AN ENTREPRENEUR? cli

KNOWLEDGE clii

RISK-TAKING clii

PLANNING... cliii

PROFESSIONALISM cliv

AFFIRMATIONS clv

KEY POINTS clvi

CHAPTER TWELVE .... **clvii**

    SELF-LOVE clvii

    WHAT IS SELF-LOVE? .... clix_Toc111570722

    SELF-LOVE VS NARCISSISM clx

    PERFECTIONISM AND ILLS clxi

    The Ills of Perfectionism clxi

    DEALING WITH PERFECTIONISM clxii

    WHY PRACTICE SELF-LOVE? clxiv

    HOW DO YOU PRACTICE SELF-LOVE? clxv

        Quit The Comparisons clxv

    Be Around People You Feel Good With clxv

    Make Room for Healthy Habits clxvii

    AFFIRMATIONS clxviii

    KEY POINTS clxix

CHAPTER THIRTEEN .... **clxx**

    MENTAL/EMOTIONAL HEALING clxx

    WHAT IS EMOTIONAL HEALING? clxx

    WHY EMOTIONAL HEALING? clxxi

    EFFECTS OF EMOTIONAL PAIN clxxii

    Anger clxxii

    Low Self-Esteem clxxiii

    Insomnia clxxiii

    STAGES OF HEALING clxxiv

    STAGE ONE: GRIEF AND DENIAL clxxv

    STAGE TWO: ANGER clxxvi

    STAGE FOUR: DEPRESSION clxxvii

STAGE FIVE: ACCEPTANCE clxxviii
POSITIVE AFFIRMATIONS FOR MENTAL HEALING clxxix
KEY POINTS clxxx

CHAPTER FOURTEEN clxxxi

YOU ARE ENOUGH clxxxi
WHAT IS SELF-WORTH? clxxxii
Confident Approach to Solving Problems clxxxiii
Realistic Expectations clxxxiv
Have Healthier Relationships clxxxiv
Resilience clxxxv
HOW TO IMPROVE YOUR SELF-WORTH clxxxvi
Come to Terms with the Positives clxxxvii
Do What You Love clxxxviii
Address Yourself With Care clxxxix
POSITIVE AFFIRMATIONS cxc
KEY POINTS cxci

Conclusion cxcii

Introduction

Dear black woman, I see you and all your work to ensure that things work out for you. I see your tears, tenacity, and drive for nothing but the exceptional. That is why I am writing this book of affirmations to encourage you.

This book contains affirmations for every stage and season. I poured myself into writing this book for you. I hope you enjoy it.

CHAPTER ONE

Beyond The Surface

"Get in touch with the depth and silence of your soul."

A lot of things have shown me how people look at reality. Small talk, probably on the bus, books, movies, and social media especially! If I say I'm not intrigued by these takes, I'd be lying because some are too crazy to be brushed aside.

Now, I'm not here to be critical about the way people have chosen to think. Everyone has the right to believe whatever they want, and there's freedom of ideology, belief, faith, and many more abstract concepts. I agree with that.

But I know I'm not the only person who will freak out whenever I hear someone say that the body has no connection with something bigger than itself or that the physical body exists on its right?

It's probably not the way you're looking at it right now. I will not start arguing with anyone about their beliefs because that will only be a severe waste of time and energy.

Even if we fail to admit it, there will always be the silent "Woah" moment in our lives. When we hear or see something out of our norm, we are in our minds like, "Woah?" And it then looks like the world replies, "Oh yeah, you haven't seen anything yet."

That is what will happen to me when I hear someone say that the physical body exists on its own. Because the concept is very sacred to me, I've had first-hand experiences that have made this concept too much of an apparent reality, only for someone else to tell me otherwise. Yeah, that's going to mess with my head for some time. Still, there's no time to dwell on the unimportant parts of life, like worrying about another person's values or opinions, especially when that person is a grown-up like you or even older.

The best anyone like me can do let you all know what it means to me and what knowing about it can do to change a lot of things about our lives.

Let's move on.

Finding out the Essence of the Spiritual Self

A lot of important things today are highly dependent on their essence. The question of essence revolves around so many things in this life. Money, fame, power, we often find ourselves asking, "what's the essence of all these?" And the same goes for what I'm about to discuss with you today.

What's the essence of the spiritual self? Why is it a thing or concept we may have to bother ourselves about? What is there to learn about it?

Finding out the essence of something may or may not change much about how a person would see such things. So even if a blockbuster movie was made, featuring all the movie stars in Hollywood about finding the essence of spirituality, a lot of people are going to enjoy the thrill and other cool stuff, but who doesn't want to get the real message, still won't.

That, however, won't discourage me from letting you know the essence of your spirituality.
But wait a sec. I haven't even told you guys what spirituality means!

How forgetful of me!

So what is spirituality?

I like how Christina Puchalski, MD, Director of the George Washington Institute for Spirituality and Health, puts it. She says;

"Spirituality is the aspect of humanity that refers to the way individuals seek and express meaning and purpose and the way they experience their connectedness to the moment, to self, to others, to nature, and the significant or sacred."

And I couldn't agree less with her. I still don't understand what that means. Alright, I'll try to do some justice to it.

In humans or most humans (let me put it that way.) There's this feeling that there's that one thing beyond our sight and even beyond our understanding responsible for whatever happens to us daily. Deja vu? Coincidence? Some people feel it's a casual event, and it's gone out the window before they even know it.

But then, some people think that something beyond the natural is responsible for what has happened!

That's quite close to what I'm looking for, you see, that urge to find a connection between yourself and some forces that you feel may be in control of your life or specific events.

Another way I look at this is that we want to find out what that one connection is between the physical and spiritual, and we want to stay plugged in for as long as we can.

There are many ways people claim to access or connect to this innermost part of themselves that they seek to find.

Some may discover that their spiritual life is intricately linked to their association with a church, temple, mosque, or synagogue. In other words, religion.

Others may pray for or seek comfort in a personal relationship with God or a higher power. For some, their spirituality is tied to specific questions they ask themselves;

Am I a good person?

What is my connection to the world ?
What is the significance of my whole existence?
What is the best way to live my life?

Yet still and enjoyable is that others seek meaning through their connections to nature or art. Like your sense of purpose, your definition of spirituality may change throughout your life, adapting to your own experiences and relationships.

How do you think you're connected to your spirituality if you think you are?

Not one for me to answer, so I'll leave that to you. Having laid a fair foundation for what spirituality is, what is its essence? Why is it that important?
Here are a few reasons why;

It defines the purpose of one's life; a lot of people are confused as to why they exist. Everyone has come to this world for a purpose, with something to achieve before they leave. No matter how "negligible" some people may see some things to be, that could be why a person was born to this earth, and getting in touch with your spiritual self, can prove very effective in helping you find your purpose in life.

Peace and Harmony: not only does spirituality promote peace and harmony between different people, but it also promotes an enabling environment for relaxation to reign within oneself. Or do you not know that battles are within the mind? Getting in touch with that spiritual self brings peace.

Promotes Love: I believe that we would not be able to love appropriately without getting in touch with our spirituality. We all know that love is beyond physical contact and romance. It entails a lot more; it is accepting and coping with the weaknesses of someone else or even yourself, having to forgive someone for a wrong they did to you. Having to make yourself uncomfortable to make another person comfortable without expecting anything in return is something one can do only when they are in touch with her spirituality. It takes more than physical attraction to do that. Trust me.

Courage: in life, people make a lot of mistakes. And some of those mistakes are meant to happen, no matter how grave. Ordinarily, we are scared of making these mistakes mainly because of the consequences we may have to face as a result of doing that. But the plain truth is this; spirituality teaches us not to be afraid of making mistakes because they're inevitable and necessary for growth. And I agree with that.

There are many reasons why humans should get in touch with our spiritual side. So much more than these just mentioned, but for space and time, I will have to conclude here and go on to other aspects of the subject of discussion.

RELIGION AND SPIRITUALITY

A lot of people tend to misunderstand religion and spirituality as meaning the same thing. I'm not saying they're entirely independent, but they're not the same.

More often than not, religion involves practicing rules, ethics, and certain beliefs in reverence to a supernatural being who may not be present but is believed to be in some unnatural way. Spirituality has to do more with yourself and your personal growth, which certain practices of religion can sometimes achieve.

Now that's where a connection comes in.

The practice of these specific laid down rules, ethics, and all that sort can help people know their spiritual selves. But that can only happen when such a person wants it and is determined enough to want to grow.

That's why we see so many people who are religious fanatics, but they're always up to no good. I hope you get what I mean; I'm not saying that people who try to get in touch with their spirituality are all good people, no one is perfect, but it's heartwarming to see those who try.

So it's good to be religious, no doubt. But there's no need to be religious when your spirit is lacking. To me, it's a total waste of time, so there's no need for it at all. But while you are religious, channel that religiosity to building up your spiritual life, and that's when you're going to enjoy it.

You know, sometimes or most times even, people are religious because they have no choice. They probably had their guardians or parents as an officer of the church or mosque and had to do the holy stuff, but their hearts weren't in sync with what they did.

Waste of youth.

EMOTIONAL HEALTH AND SPIRITUALITY

There's also a connection between mental health and spiritual health. You notice that many practices recommended for building up spirituality are similar to those recommended for improving emotional well-being because the two are connected, as do all aspects of well-being; emotional and spiritual well-being influence one another and overlap.

Once again, I'd like to reiterate that they're not the same. Spirituality is mostly about finding a meaningful connection with something much bigger than yourself, which can result in positive emotions, such as peace, awe, contentment, gratitude, forgiveness, and many other virtues. Meanwhile, emotional health is about cultivating a positive state of mind, which can broaden your outlook to recognize and incorporate a connection to something larger than yourself.

Thus, emotions and spirituality are different but linked, deeply integrated. Thus, emotions and spirituality are distinct but linked, deeply integrated.

IMPACTS OF SPIRITUALITY ON MENTAL HEALTH

The idea of spirituality as a whole has different meanings for different people, and spiritual beliefs are as many as the people who practice them. But, despite the difference in these beliefs, they all have something in common. They all affect our mental health.

Spirituality affects our mental health in so many ways. Spirituality mainly concerns your belief or a sense of purpose and meaning. It gives you a sense of value or worth in your life.

And like I've said before, contrary to what many people might think, spirituality and religion are not the same. But they indeed have a connection. You can be spiritual without belonging to a specific religion. Religious people abide by a particular faith and may be connected with specific groups or traditions, while spirituality is primarily a journey embarked on by only you.

So how does spirituality affect our mental health? Spirituality has a significant influence on a high percentage of human decisions. It makes people probe into the nature of their being, the physical life, and the spiritual, which the bare eyes cannot behold.

Spirituality can help deal with stress by giving you a sense of peace, purpose, and forgiveness, so it often becomes more important in times of emotional stress or illness.

As much as spirituality can do good, it can also be detrimental to certain people, and we'll find out sooner.

To put it in a way that anyone can quickly grasp, here are some of the several ways that spirituality can be of support to our mental health:

You may feel a higher sense of purpose, peace, hope, and meaning.
You may experience better confidence, self-esteem, and self-control.
It can help you make sense of your experiences in life.
When unwell, it can help you feel inner strength and result in faster recovery.
Those in a spiritual community may have more support.
You may work at better relationships with yourself and others.

In addition, many people with a mental illness get a sense of faith and hope by talking with a religious or spiritual leader.

And the fact that some mental illnesses present themselves as times when people question their value or purpose in a way that leaves them feeling pessimistic and hopeless makes it extremely helpful to include spirituality in treating mental health difficulties.

Having said this, how can spirituality be detrimental to certain people, and what set of people are they in particular? Even if we do not admit it, the truth remains that we live in a ruthless world with so many people up to no good out there. That is why some people may take advantage of emotionally vulnerable people while pretending to support their spirituality. If you're emotionally vulnerable, you can be more easily convinced to participate in harmful activities to improve your spirituality. Meanwhile, you're just being used or extorted. Concerning this, we must note that the spirituality here is not true; anyone should be able to spot what is fake and what is real. As for me, the yardstick is that true spirituality shouldn't cause me discomfort either spiritually or physically. I need to feel at ease to know I'm on the right track.

IMPROVING SPIRITUAL HEALTH

We need to talk about how we can improve our spiritual health. Having spoken about what it entails, its importance, and others, it all comes down to how we can make this spirituality work effectively for us.

And how can anyone make anything work more effectively for them without improvement? I honestly do not have an answer to that.

Different approaches work differently for other people. But the essential part is that you do what gives you the most joy and comfort.

These are some of the ideas one can use to improve their spiritual health;

Discover the things that make you feel alive, joyful, loved, and in unison with the rhythm of your soul.
Dedicate part of your day doing community service.
Read inspirational books.
Try meditating.
Take a walk outdoors.
Pray – alone or with a group.
Practice yoga.
Play your favorite sport.
Dedicate quiet time to yourself.

In concluding this section, I'd like to add that a spiritual health evaluation is sometimes necessary as a part of any mental health assessment. It is because mental issues like depression and substance abuse can be a sign or result of a spiritual void in your life. Therefore understanding the distinction between a spiritual crisis and a mental health issue is essential to getting to the root of the problem and finding the solution as well.

Do you see how the concept of spirituality cuts through every aspect of human life? I tell you for sure that growth is inevitable when you get in touch with that aspect of your life.

AFFIRMATIONS FOR SPIRITUALITY

1. I will not be critical of the way people have chosen to live their lives
2. I believe that there's more to life than the physical and social interactions
3. I cannot be 100% in control of my life
4. I've come to this world for a purpose
5. I have to find peace within myself.
6. I believe that it takes more than physical touch and romance to love
7. My mistakes are not who I am
8. I fear no mistakes.
9. I'm going to learn from my mistakes.
10. I believe religion and spirituality mean different things
11. I will not be oblivious to the connection between religion and spirituality
12. I am going to combine religion and spirituality to my advantage
13. I will not be a religious fanatic and be spiritually empty.
14. I have great value for my emotional health
15. I will channel my spirituality to making the right decisions and doing the right things

16. I will not take advantage of people who are emotionally vulnerable in the name of improving their spiritual life.
17. This cruel world will not allow me to be taken advantage of.
18. In practicing spirituality, I shouldn't have to feel discomfort.
19. I will embrace the connection I share with all life on this Earth.
20. I am always open to having a new experience of reality for myself
21. Little by little, I am connecting with my true purpose on Earth.
22. My age doesn't have anything to do with who I am or what I do; I am infinite.
23. I am connected with my soul every time of the day.
24. The universe hands me whatever I need at the right time.
25. I am a spiritual being have an earthly experience
26. I can tap into the abundance of the universe
27. I believe that whatever happens to me happens for my good.
28. The divine energy flows through me every day
29. I am worth whatever time I need to nourish my soul
30. I am open to loving my spirit more
31. I will always lend my ears to the voice of encouragement inside me
32. I am consciously and constantly aligned with my spiritual self
33. I am going to allow the universe to work through me
34. All of my thoughts, words, and actions are inspired by the divine
35. I am powerful enough to deal with negativity.

KEY POINTS

1. There's always more to life than what we see with our physical eyes.

2. Nobody has a similar experience of spirituality; people experience spirituality differently.
3. Every human being has a purpose in life. Some may or may not live long enough to achieve it.
4. Peace within should be your priority.
5. One has to be wary of how people describe spirituality to look.
6. Religion and spirituality do not mean the same thing but can be used together to improve the quality of our lives.
7. Improving our spiritual health is key to improving our mental health as well.

CHAPTER TWO

SELF AWARENESS

"It takes courage...to endure the sharp pains of self-discovery rather than choose to take the dull pain of unconsciousness that would last the rest of our lives."
-Marianne Williamson

Let me tell you a little story about myself.

It was my eighteenth birthday anniversary that day, and the day was almost over when my Dad called me into his room.

We were alone in the room, and he said to me,

"Son, I have a gift for you."

He then held my shoulders and spoke.

"This will be the greatest gift you have ever received. It is the key to your guaranteed success, and you have no choice but to use it well enough to yield the desired results, except you want to prove to me that bringing you up was a waste of time. Am I clear?"

I was perplexed. But I nodded slowly as my heart trembled in anticipation of whatever gift he had for me. I didn't want to be optimistic that the gift held the key to my success. Parents possess the art of exaggeration, so I had to keep the excitement low.

My Dad went into his drawer and slowly brought out something. I couldn't see it because he turned his back on me. And then the atmosphere began to feel like Hollywood as he began to shake the dust out of whatever he held.

He glanced at it and then turned to me, holding the object to his back. He walked toward me and said,

"You must use this every day and treat this with care if you seek good results."

It was a book, and the book's title was my name.
My Dad told me the book contained all I needed to know about myself and how I'm supposed to live my life according to it.

It seemed like a joke, but when I read the book and religiously followed the instructions on how I was supposed to love my life, that was when I realized that I could write books, and that's when I became the best writer in the world, winning five consecutive Pulitzer awards for writing and eventually becoming the wealthiest man on the globe after selling millions of copies of the books I've written.

What a story! Or most of you must be saying, what a lie!

But it seemed like an exciting and credible story, didn't it? Or at what point did you stop believing it?

Most definitely the point where I said I won 5 Pulitzer awards and became the wealthiest man globally. And you'll be like, oh yeah, this guy's making this all up.

Because yes! I concede that I'm making this all up because I've got something to point out to you.

Most people don't understand that they have to know themselves. Or let me put it this way: some people think they should know themselves because, why not? Am I not the one? Why shouldn't I know myself? Completely failing to realize that it is possible for them not to know themselves entirely and how they're wired!

Before we continue, I feel like there's a question that most readers would have in their minds. Maybe they don't have it per se, but it just takes a little jolting, and if I bring it to their attention, they're going to realize that they need to have an answer to it to understand what's going on here entirely.

According to the story I made up, I was 18, and my father still felt the need to give me a book about myself. Don't you think that's strange? I'm 18 years old; for heaven's sake, why would my father think that the best gift he'd give to me is a book about myself? At 18, what don't I already know about myself that I need a book to tell me?

Well, the truth is, I don't think we completely know ourselves enough to live life the way we ought to. And when that stage of self-realization comes in our lives, we must find out who we are and what we want.

Don't ask your Dad; that's just fiction. Even your friends would know you better than your Dad. It's your journey and yours alone. The path to self-determination is lonely, and that's how it's meant to be.

No one has the power to know you more than you, and if you don't know yourself, there might be a lot of complications along the way if you don't act fast enough.

WHY DO I NEED TO KNOW MYSELF?

I know, right? Why do we need to know ourselves more than we already know before? I mean, isn't it possible to live with the information we already have about ourselves and keep going on and on?

Why does life have to get this complicated?

Well, it's left for anyone to do as they wish with their lives anyway. It's a matter of choice, not anyone else's choice, but mine and yours to live however they want to.

But I still think it's fair to share my opinion on why we should strive to know ourselves. You know, to fulfill all righteousness. The work has to be complete. I'm going to do just that.

Humans spend a lot of time worrying about our relationships with others and how they feel or think about us. But, the truth is the only relationship that matters in life is the one you have with yourself. Even if you're born twins, you will not die as one.

You're the only one going to be there for yourself when no one else can; it is only you, from the cradle to the grave. Not to sound selfish, but to emphasize why you need to know yourself.

These are some reasons why it is essential to know yourself.

Self-Love

If you know yourself, the good, the bad, and the ugly, that's a perfect starting point to accepting who you are - exactly as you are. It's going to feel like a challenge, trying to get aspects of your character that you're not a fan of, such as laziness and the sort.

However, if that is already a part of you and you've tried hard to change but cannot, it is important to honor that instead of denying it. It'll still be there, even if you decline it.

Applying a different approach could help too. Instead of trying to stop being lazy, learning to see the benefits of laziness, enjoying it, and not allowing it to work against you will enable you to embrace it as part of who you are and to, therefore, love it. You can move from love to nurturing, growing, developing, thriving, and flourishing.

Independence

When you know yourself, it makes you independent of how others feel about you. If you know what works for you, what is the best for you, and, therefore, what isn't - it becomes irrelevant what others might think and advise.
Like I said earlier, no one can know you more than you know yourself. You are the expert of your being. You are in charge of your thoughts and actions, and you are your personality.

Independence and self-awareness can also be linked to self-confidence. Thus, knowing who you are and what you stand for in life can help to give you a strong sense of self-confidence. Copy that?

Clear Decision Making

It is common knowledge that with knowledge comes insight and confidence, which are practical tools in decision-making (for both simple and complicated choices) to make it much more manageable. No one can doubt that when there's a level of understanding or insight about something, making decisions concerning such things becomes a piece of cake. So when we know ourselves to a great extent, making decisions that pertain to us wouldn't be much of a problem, and there's not going to be so much doubt about it.

There's this theory by Dr. Marriet Johnson that we all speak two languages: the language of the heart and that of the head. If they are aligned, it becomes effortless to make a decision. But if they're not, it just depends on your mood and what you think is right or wrong. And making decisions depending on your present mood can be very dangerous because attitudes can change in seconds. You don't want to make decisions based on fluctuating standards, do you? She further gives an example;

You are about to purchase a house and find one that meets all your requirements. However, something about the place makes you uneasy. You are unsure what it is, but it doesn't feel okay.

Having two contrasting dialogues in your head makes everything complicated. Today, your head tells you what to do, and you want to buy the house; tomorrow, it's your heart telling you not to go on with purchasing the home. Syncing your head and heart will give clarity, which supports easy decision-making.

These are a few of the many reasons why you need to know yourself. I don't know what else will convince you if you don't find any of these reasons convincing enough. I've done all I can for now.

So how do you know yourself?

How do you know anything at all? Pretty sure a vast percentage of us have gone through the process of trying to learn something, in one way or the other.
It could be in school, at the workplace, at home in front of the computer on YouTube, so many ways!

What are you trying to do there? You're trying to know something, and what are you doing to get that knowledge? You're learning! Simple!

That answers the question of how you know yourself. You know yourself through learning about yourself; the real question that should be full of content is how do you remember about yourself? That's where all the answers lie. Stick around, it's going to be an exciting ride, and you're surely going to go home with something you've never had before.

LEARNING ABOUT YOURSELF

Knowing your true self is one of the essential powers you can possess. When you know who you are, you always know what you need to do instead of seeking validation from others. It helps you to bypass the frustration caused by putting time into the wrong things.

Of course, life isn't a bed of roses and is supposed to be full of trial and error, but self-awareness lets you discover the best areas to experiment with.

Good knowledge of self will help you build confidence that cannot be shattered, and you will gain a deeper meaning of your purpose in life and eventually impact the world.

So, what is the secret to knowing oneself? Come with me as I explore tips to help you better understand yourself.

Be Still

You cannot and will not be able to discover yourself until you take the time to be still. Never underestimate the power of peace; many people don't have any idea of themselves because any silence scares them; all they want is the noise, the buzz; it's too sorrowful to be alone with all their flaws staring back at them. They always want the noise to overshadow their weaknesses.

But it isn't until you go to a quiet place and assess yourself while being completely honest with yourself that you will be able to see every aspect of your life clearly —the good, the bad, and the ugly.

Be quiet and discover who you are.

Distinguish Between Who You Are And Who You Want To Be

I understand that you already have a set idea of who you desperately want to be, but you might want to sit back and ask yourself, is this really who I am? Or are these expectations I've set for myself the ones I should meet? That picture you've already painted of yourself in your head might not be who you were designed to be. Knowing who you are will finally see where you and your specific gifts fit into the bigger picture. You can always be better than that person you desperately want to be.

And although there are many points along your journey to help you discover yourself, one of the best ways to start is to take a personality test. You can take it more than once, especially when it's been a while since you last took the previous one. And even if these self-evaluations aren't perfect, they do pinpoint your top areas of strengths or weaknesses, so you can focus on the change you were meant to bring into the world.

I tell you again; you can be so much better than that painting you already made in your head, so much better.

Find Out Your Strengths And Weaknesses

It might be the most challenging step in discovering who you are, but it's one you must take. No doubt, it takes a lot of trial and error to find out what you're good at, and you don't have to give up before you've made more than enough attempts, but you must realize that knowing when to quit is a gift that everyone needs to learn. You think leaving is not an option, no, no, no, not true.

You have to quit when you've put in so much time, and all your efforts fall shy.

Now, what is the measure for "so much time?" No one else but you can decide that, at least, you should know yourself up to that extent. But I want you to know that there's a big difference between quitting correctly and giving up. When you quit correctly, you're making room for something better. When I say something better, I mean something beneficial to you.

Take the hint when your actions begin to drain you rather than produce more passion and increase your drive to do more. That's a good sign it is time to focus elsewhere. Your strengths will show you who you indeed are, that's for sure. So build on them.

Follow Your Passion

The following passion of any kind is a good thing, and that's one of the aspects of your life that you need to pay attention to when it comes. The reason is that it shows an area of your life on which you need to focus more attention and resources.

If we're also talking about following your passion for work, that's a good one. And if it is having more passion for life, it's also a good thing.

Focus more on passion; I see passion as a gold mine because it makes you understand yourself better, allowing you to make a significant impact. Passion births effort and continuous effort produces results that produce a more profound discovery of your true self.

AFFIRMATIONS FOR SELF AWARENESS

1. I will embark on a journey to self-awareness and discovery.
2. No one knows me better than myself
3. I will focus less on what others think or say about me.

4. I will focus more on the relationship I have with myself
5. I will accept rather than deny who I truly am.
6. I will always try to see the silver lining in the dark clouds.
7. I love myself
8. I take control of my words and actions
9. I am my personality.
10. I am confident in who I am and all I stand for.
11. I will not base my decision-making on fluctuating standards.
12. I will always be ready to learn how to be self-aware.
13. I will not seek the validation of others.
14. I am bold enough to be still and face my flaws
15. I will not rely on the weaknesses of others to make me feel better
16. I will be completely honest to myself no matter the circumstances
17. I can be better than whoever I desperately want to be.
18. I will not give up easily, but I will know when to quit.
19. I will discover my strengths and build upon them.
20. I will follow my passion always
21. I will take advantage of any opportunity life offers me to make an impact
22. The journey to self-awareness is never-ending, and I am willing to go all for it.
23. I become aware of my innate talent every day
24. I continue to discover more of what makes me unique by the day
25. Being self-aware is one of my top priorities, and I work towards it every day
26. I always get to understand myself better every day
27. I will always allow myself to be myself no matter what it costs.
28. I am committed to finding out who I am and what I can achieve
29. I carefully monitor how I talk and think to myself every day

30. Whatever benefits me, I recognize and begin to nurture them
31. I know what I want in my life, and I work towards achieving them
32. I am striving to be fully aware of my feelings every day
33. If it's ever going to be, it's always up to me
34. It is one of my greatest desires to live each day fully aware of myself

KEY POINTS

1. No one can know yourself better than you do.
2. Learn to accept yourself the way you are sometimes.
3. Your improvement never ends.
4. Never rely on others' opinions about you.
5. Never make decisions based on your present mood.
6. You don't always need the noise.
7. You might not be cut out to be who you want to be. Accept that.
8. Forget about what you cannot do and build on your strengths
9. Your passion is your gold mine; follow it consistently.
10. The journey to self-awareness does not end.

CHAPTER THREE

SEXUALITY

"We have the means and knowledge to achieve universal sexual and reproductive health and rights. Meaningful progress is possible, it is affordable and it is vital."
~Ann M. Starrs, Co-chair Guttmacher-Lancet Commission.

In my book Spiritual Self-Care For Black Women, I talked a lot about sexuality and how it could be linked to spirituality. I know quite alright that the topic of sexuality can be vast, and that is why I'm writing about it again. In my previous book, I talked about many things; a brief history of human sexuality, a woman's sexuality, sexual development, puberty in girls, the concepts of honor killings, shame, and wrong teachings. Also, we could differentiate between sexual identity, sexual orientation, and sexual behavior, know the types of sexual orientation and gender identities, how sexuality affects spirituality: the link between the two concepts, and how to sync your spirituality with sex.

This time, you and I will be looking at sexual problems in women and living above the stigma of STDs. As we begin this emotional but enlightening ride, I encourage you to brace yourself. You're a strong black woman; always remember that.

Sexual Problems In Women

When talking about sex, I believe it encompasses both the pleasurable aspect and the, what should I call it, not-so-pleasurable aspect? It is no news that women's sexuality was once considered taboo to be spoken about. Still, women are changing the narrative worldwide now, and I believe this book and the rest of my books on sexuality will catalyze this cause.

Quickly, we shall be looking at the sexual problems in women but not without having an understanding of the sexual response cycle. Every human has a sexual cycle, both men and women, and all stages are passed through at different rates. In a situation where one step is missed, there is a problem. I'll briefly speak on the four:

Excitement Phase: This phase is also called desire, where a woman has this urge to engage in sexual activity like a charge in her body, prompting her to be responsive. It comes with quickened heartbeats and breathing and also flushed skin.

Plateau Phase or Arousal Phase: Immediately a woman enters the excitement phase, what could lead her to the next step largely depends on sexual stimulation. How she's touched or touches, what she hears and sees, the sort. In the arousal stage, the vagina secretes fluids in preparation for intercourse. It also expands while the clitoris enlarges and the nipples become erect.

Orgasm: This stage marks the peak of a woman's sexual response cycle, which has the muscles of the vagina contracting rhythmically and resulting in a mix of different emotions, with pleasure usually the first. It is also the climax stage.

Resolution: This is the last stage after a woman has successfully climaxed. It features her body relaxing, her clitoris, vagina, and nipples all relaxing and returning to their unaroused states.

As I have earlier stated, my dear black woman, any omission of these stages by your body will result in a sexual problem, and how do you know there's an omission? How d'you realize that there's a dysfunction in your sex life?

Symptoms such as spasms of vaginal muscles, absence of the excitement phase, experiencing pain during intercourse, etc., are a few of the numerous ways to know you have sexual dysfunction. If you experience any of these, my first advice to you is that you remain calm and brave as we continue. It should be easy for you to do; you are, after all, a black woman. In this book, types, causes, and solutions to female sexual problems will be discussed.

Female Sexual Problems

Dyspareunia: This is the abnormal pain you experience before, during, or after sexual intercourse.

Anorgasmia: This can be very frustrating for a woman who can feel excited but cannot experience orgasm and may have her desiring sex less. It is the term for delayed or infrequent orgasms. It's also the inability to have powerful orgasms or even just an orgasm.

Lack of sexual desire: A widespread problem in men and women. It stops the sexual response cycle before it even gets the chance to start, taking away any desire a man or woman would feel for their partner. At times, it can be temporary and ongoing at other times.

Sexual Problems can be very upsetting for men and women and can hinder sexual satisfaction, so it is trite that having known the types, we should understand the causes of these dysfunctions.

Causes Of Female Sexual Problems

Physical Causes: Gynecologic conditions such as vaginismus which causes vaginal muscle spasms, vaginitis, endometriosis, and other pelvic disorders, can make intercourse unpleasant.

Certain medications can also affect sexual functioning. Selective Serotonin-Reuptake Inhibitor (SSRI) group of antidepressants and chemotherapy may reduce your sex drive and affect your hormone levels. I used to know a woman whose name I cannot mention for privacy purposes. She was on antidepressants for quite a long time and, at the same time, was seeking solutions to a sexual dysfunction she had. The doctor diagnosed and found the antidepressants to be the cause. While this may affect some people, it may not affect others, so it's always best to seek professional help when you need to be on medications.

Hormonal imbalance may also be a cause of sexual dysfunction in women. My dear black woman, like it or not, your body is bound to go through several changes. Pregnancy, Menopause, and surgery are significant triggers of hormonal changes, and where there's an imbalance of hormones in your body, conditions such as vaginal dryness may surface, making sex painful to experience.

Other physical causes such as sexually transmitted diseases, fatigue, alcohol and drug intake, chronic diseases such as kidney diseases, heart diseases, radiation therapy, history of sexual and other types of abuse, and contrasting beliefs about sex may also hinder an extraordinary sexual experience.

Diagnosis Of Female Sexual Problems

To become fully in charge of your sexuality, you, my beautiful black woman, must be committed to seeing that things are right in your life, including your sexual health. Be vigilant and observant. When you notice anything unusual during sexual intercourse, I am here to plead and advise you to seek professional help.

When a sexual problem persists for weeks, it's only fitting that you stop ignoring or letting procrastination get the best of you and go for a checkup. Starting treatments on time can and has proven to go a long way in treating many illnesses. While some symptoms may persist for weeks, others may require immediate attention due to the advancement of the symptoms. Overall, it would help if you didn't hesitate to seek medical attention no matter how mild you may consider the signs to be. You're a brave woman, and I believe you can do this.

During diagnosis and tests, provide health care professionals with information regarding any underlying health condition you may have. In the absence of any, ensure to be as honest as you can with them. Also, please provide them with information about whether you're on medications or not and what medications you're on. Your gynecologist will perform a physical or pelvic examination and may refer you to other specialists for consultations.

Blood tests, imaging, and papsmear tests may also be carried out. You may be required to speak to a relationship counselor or mental health professional for psychological cases. You don't have to panic when seeking help, and always remember Lily Collins' words: "Asking for help is never a sign of weakness. It's one of the bravest things you can do. And it can save your life."

Treatment Of Female Sexual Problems

I think the first step to treating sexual problems is the acceptance of them. Many people like to live in denial about certain things in their lives to avoid "depression," but the natural depression comes when they find out it's too late. I wouldn't like this to be your fate, my beautiful black woman. You come first in everything, and that includes your sexual health.

When diagnosed with a dysfunction, some problems require you to wait it out, but if this isn't your case, you have to swing into action immediately.

There are some physical solutions to try out;

Arousal Techniques: Create time for yourself and your partner, free of every distraction. Increase stimulation and arousal by watching erotic videos or reading erotic books, masturbating, and using sensual massages.

Trying out different sexual techniques and discussing your sexual fantasies with your partner can help to boost sex and help you relax. A warm bath before sex is also good to try out, leaving you feeling relaxed.

Clitoral Therapy Device: This is an approved treatment device by the U.S Food and Drug Administration (FDA) for treating women with sexual dysfunction, particularly problems with arousal and orgasms. It increases lubrication when placed over the clitoris and enables a woman to orgasm.

Lubricants: If you experience vaginal dryness, vaginal lubricants should be the first thing you try. They do not need a prescription and can be found in stores. Scientists and I, likewise, recommend water-based products. Oil-based products are not the best choices as they might cause latex condoms to break. Trust me on this one.

Counseling: As discussed earlier, some sexual dysfunctions can be caused by trauma, stress, or other psychologically related causes. Using the services of a mental health therapist can go a long way in boosting your sex life. The therapist or counselor would help you identify negative attitudes and past traumatic experiences such as abuse and rape and teach you ways of overcoming these negative thoughts and experiences. The process can be painfully slow depending on how adverse the causes are, but believe me, if you're keen on overcoming these negative experiences, you will.

Surgery: Some sexual dysfunctions cannot be cured by physical solutions or psychotherapy, and in such cases, surgery is required. Specific issues like tumors and cysts require surgery for an improved sexual experience.

Prevention Of Female Sexual Problems

I've carefully listed a few methods to follow to prevent sexual problems from occurring within yourself as a woman or between you and your partner. Research has proven them helpful in curbing the spread of sexual problems in persons.

Communication: This is one of the secrets to a healthy relationship and healthy sex life. If you have underlying health conditions, be truthful to your partner and seek medical solutions. If the sex with your partner feels different, they should be the first person you talk to.

Meditations, Regular Exercises, Rest, and a Healthy Diet are principal to being relaxed and boosting your hormones.

Live a healthy lifestyle. Avoid smoking and alcohol. Also, attend regular and recommended checkups and health screenings.

LIVING ABOVE THE STIGMA OF STDS

Let's be brutally honest with ourselves; the names are pretty scary: Chlamydia, Gonorrhea, Syphilis, Human papillomavirus, Human Immunodeficiency Virus, Herpes, Genital warts, Crabs, and Trichomonas, to name a few.

Most are even almost impossible to spell, let alone be voiced. But the complicated phonics or spellings are the least of what people are concerned about when it comes to discussing sexually transmitted diseases (STDs), and no matter how long these STDs have been in existence, a lot of stigmas still hover around them.

Honesty Is Key

Just like some people hide their COVID-19 diagnosis from the public for fear of being judged and shamed, so do people diagnosed with STDs. If you ever feel alone because of an

STD you're diagnosed with; I'm here to encourage you and let you know that no matter what you think, you should never have to lie about your condition. Understand that people will always talk and want to stigmatize you for having an STD, but they only penetrate you if you permit them. We'll get to a point where STDs no longer have to be associated with words such as "promiscuous" or "unclean," and you, my black woman, would be standing tall and proud by then.

Anyone can get an STI. It's even more common than people realize. If people catch infections just by handshakes, why should conditions from sex be more shameful?

Helping Yourself And Others

One mistake people make is believing that since STIs are very common, talking about them would be easy. In truth, it isn't. We've talked about why people shy away from the topic or admit being optimistic about it, but there's no way you'll help others if you see STDs as a form of a death sentence. People live their best lives with STDs and STIs, and so should you, my dear black woman.

I want you to raise your head high and promise to be everything but sad and in constant denial. You're owning up to everything you've passed through and arming yourself to help others.

A step to helping others is by being educated and knowing facts about STDs. That way, your fears would be allayed, and your confidence boosted. Joining support groups or creating one that talks about sexual problems and ways of overcoming them can also be helpful. It gives hope to people as well as yourself and is a safe space for meeting people going through similar circumstances and knowing their stories.

The next one I'm about to say might be absurd and straight to the point, but I'll say it either way. Date people with the same diagnosis as they would understand you better, and you would feel more at peace with them. Joining dating sites set up expressly to match people with STIs can speed things up and make you feel more at ease.

Talking about it on time also helps, including being honest with people, and your partner. If you recently started dating, you should be open and honest with them about your sexual health status before sexual intercourse, but only if you deem them to be worth it.

Importance of Breaking The Stigma

My dear black woman, I understand the stigma of STDs and STIs and how the fear of being tested positive might be so paralyzing, but I need you to realize that what is more dreadful is dying in silence.

If you feel something's wrong with your body, go for a checkup. If you think you feel okay, go for a checkup too. Either way, always go for checkups frequently. Some STIs are asymptomatic, while others may take years before manifesting physical symptoms, which would have been too late. Equip yourself with new information every day and live healthily.

Affirmations For A Positive Sexual Health

1. I am confident in my sexual life
2. I can do all I desire with my body
3. I will entertain only positive thoughts on my sexuality
4. Communicating with my partner about my sexual desires is straightforward.
5. I glow with sexual energy
6. Sharing my deepest sexual fantasies with my partner is natural.
7. I am worthy of the love I receive from my partner
8. I am safe and satisfied in my bed.
9. Sexual intercourse is fun for me.
10. Exploring my body makes me feel happy.
11. I have a healthy sex life.
12. My orgasms are frequent and powerful.
13. My partner can sexually arouse me and make me feel desired.
14. My genitals are entirely healthy.
15. I am willing to listen to my partner's sexual insecurities.
16. I am conscious of seeking ways to boost sexual experiences with my partner.
17. Rejection by a potential sexual partner will not make me feel lowly of myself.
18. My libido is alive!
19. I am a masterpiece, and so is my body.
20. I see sex as sacred and honor my partner.
21. I refuse to avoid my sexual desires but rather embrace them.
22. I feel no pain during sexual intercourse.
23. My partner makes me experience sexual pleasure and makes me feel loved.
24. I am in charge of my thoughts and feelings.
25. I am a natural at pleasing my partner and myself.

26. I know how to guide my partner to please me better.
27. My body is strong enough to fend off any sickness.
28. I am a sexy black woman.
29. My relationship with my partner is healthy and meaningful.
30. I am sexually satisfied.
31. I am constantly exploring and embracing my sexual desires
32. My sex life is a priority as it is necessary for my health and stress relief
33. I will be open to my partner about things that I enjoy and the things I do not
34. I only engage in passionate relationships while setting healthy boundaries
35. I am in complete control of my sexual thought, desires, and behaviors.

Key Points

1. The four sexual cycles women go through are the excitement phase, the arousal phase, orgasm, and resolution.
2. Symptoms of sexual dysfunction include unusual pain before, during, or after intercourse, spasms of the vaginal muscles, and inability to be sexually aroused.
3. Men and women should understand the causes of sexual dysfunction to know what to do.
4. Some physical causes of female sexual problems are gynecologic conditions, SSRI group antidepressants, STDs, chronic diseases, and hormonal imbalance.
5. Never ignore anything unusual going on in your body. If such a problem persists, seek professional help.
6. Being brave involves going for regular checkups.
7. Treatment of female sexual problems includes clitoral therapy devices, counseling, arousal techniques, lubricants, and in dire cases, surgery.

8. Some sexual dysfunctions can be prevented by living healthy lifestyles.
9. No one is immune to an STI. Be truthful about yours.
10. Joining or creating support groups, dating people with the same diagnosis, and talking about it helps you overcome the negative emotions of STDs.
11. Many STIs are asymptomatic, hence the need for regular health checkups.

CHAPTER FOUR

WORKPLACE

"There's no magic formula for great company culture. The key is just to treat your staff how you would like to be treated."
- Richard Branson, Founder of Virgin Group

If we're to be honest with ourselves, having to count the top 3 most important places in our lives, I don't think there'd be any way our places won't make it to the list for obvious reasons. If the place I go to make money to survive isn't essential, I wonder what other places will be. The White House? Some people could say so, but I'm not sure I'll be one of them.

Defining the workplace may seem absurd because the name already explains itself; nevertheless, I'd still like to determine what a workplace is.

In simple terms, a workplace is where a person performs jobs or tasks for an employer or himself, as the case may be. Workplaces vary from industries and can be inside a building or situated outdoors. They can also be mobile, and some people may have to work in different locations on various days. Still, technology has enabled people to work virtually without going to the office.

I will briefly explain the types of workplaces for the sake of knowing them and for the sake of distinction.

OFFICE

The office is a common, if not the most common type of workplace in the world right now, where employees of a company perform various tasks from a centralized location. Offices can take different forms and fashion. A company's office can be a whole complex, a single building, a compartment in a shared facility, or a section of a co-working unit. There are also what we call co-working sites. It's like a recourse for smaller businesses or companies who prefer to focus on their employees and customers first before their workplace. (Who knows, you might need that knowledge somewhere else.)

Home Office

Certain businesses do not need people to perform jobs or tasks in a centralized location and can benefit mainly from allowing their employees to work remotely. The necessary software, equipment, and training are available for employees who do their jobs wherever they might be. Some people could have a designated room in their home with a desk and computer to perform their work.

Flexible work schedules should be drafted and incorporated for a smooth-running business to ensure everyone works optimally. Provisions can also be made for staff who works remotely.

Distribution or Factory Center

People work in distribution centers in various industries, especially the food, apparel, electronics, and automobile industries. They are most likely to be located near the business's corporate office rather than separate locations, which is also possible in some cases.

Factory workers make the final product in the production line, while employees from the distribution center sort products sent to stores or customers.

Farm or Outdoor Location

As much as many industries require people to work in factories and distribution centers, some also need people to work outdoors! This set of people includes farmers, environmental scientists, park rangers, construction workers, law enforcement officers, and electricians; the list goes on.

I think these guys work the hardest because, unlike others who get to work indoors, protected from harsh weather conditions, these guys have to work no matter the weather condition.

Store

Various stores include supermarkets, boutiques, grocery stores, shopping malls, etc. The employees usually work indoors and often directly interact with customers. All stores are different, and factors warranting these differences include size, geographic needs, and location.

PURPOSE OF THE WORKPLACE

Workplaces serve different purposes depending on the type. But in general, they help businesses deliver their products or services to consumers efficiently. To further break these purposes down, corporate team members use their place of work as an avenue to collaborate and develop new ideas for manufacturing products and providing services for their customers. Businesses use factories to manufacture their products and distribution centers to organize the shipment of the product to retail stores or to the consumer. Stores exist for consumers to purchase products by giving a space for customers to see the product physically.

It's like a hierarchy of purposes for the workplace as they work hand in hand to achieve a specific aim.

Having spoken much about the workplace in literal terms, I want us to recognize that beyond those buildings and structures we just talked about, there's another definition. To me, the most important one. Which I call and we all know as the "Employee."

Oh! You probably thought I was going to talk about buildings forever. Oh no, I'm not. It will focus on what I think is far more critical than structures.

People!

It shouldn't come as a shock, or does it? We'd entirely agree that without the people, or should I say, the people who are capable enough, whatever structure exists would be outright useless. Don't we?

Or we could also say that these people would not be able to work effectively if these structures were not put in place, right? But systems do not fall from the sky, do they? I'm probably asking many questions now, but I can't help it because I'm trying to point out the truth!

The structures we may feel are so crucial for the human resource to work on are put in place by humans themselves! This is why the employee or employer if you put it that way (to me, they're all employees because even the employer is working for himself, which makes him an employee to himself), should always be at the forefront of concern. As we continue in this discussion, I'd like to expose you to a few things you can do to make the workplace a conducive one for you which would entail you knowing how to treat your fellow employees, recognizing your worth even when people want to intentionally be blind to it, taking note of the red flags, and also recognizing when to call it quits.

Hang in there!

WORKPLACE STRUGGLES

Not going to lie; this is an extensive issue. As vast as the whole of Asia if you ask me. As confined as the concept of the term "workplace" is, no one should be fooled to believe that everything that goes on there revolves around work only. The workplace is another world on its own. When you leave your home for work, it's like walking into another life where almost everything, the good, the bad, and the ugly, happens.

Real struggles go on in various workplaces. Efforts that not everyone knows about keep people up late at night, force people to take their own lives, and some struggles even go with some people to their graves!

There's a lot people have to endure for so many years that it even turns to some toxic sort of enjoyment because they don't want to lose their jobs, and it's unfortunate to say that as a black woman, some of these experiences may not be new to you. But we all hope to change the narrative, rewrite the story, and lend our voices, however loud they will be.

Everyone should know what goes on. Yeah, most people have an idea, but a lot of people still don't; they're probably too young and haven't gotten a job to know these things, but most of them will one day. They have to know what to expect and how to manage whatever comes their way, don't they?

Very well then, let's begin.

Sexual Harassment

Workplace sexual harassment is defined by The United States Equal Employment Opportunity Commission (EEOC) as "unwelcome sexual advances, requests for sexual favors, and other verbal or physical conduct of a sexual nature ... when this conduct explicitly or implicitly affects an individual's employment, unreasonably interferes with an individual's work performance, or creates an intimidating, hostile, or offensive work environment."
They then went further to say;

"The challenged conduct must be unwelcome in that the employee did not solicit or incite it, and that the employee considered the conduct as undesirable or offensive."

"Particularly when the alleged harasser may have some reason (e.g., prior consensual relationship) to think that the advances will be condoned, it is important for the victim to communicate that the conduct is unwelcome."

Quite a lengthy definition involving specific ups and downs, but we all know the core of it, don't we? It shouldn't even be news to anyone above 18 to be modest. It happens everywhere!

Sexual harassment includes quite a wide range of actions, from verbal transgressions to sexual abuse or assault.

And although the victims are usually more women, we cannot rule out that men are sexually harassed too! In fact, throughout the United States, 21% of victims are men! That's, anyway, to make us understand that it can go both ways.

There's also what is called, Sexual Bribery, which is the demand of sex, any sexual activity, or other sex-related activity for a promise of a raise in work status or pay. This usually happens in an employment setting where a sexual relationship with a superior is made an explicit or implied condition for obtaining/retaining employment or its benefits.

Things like this happen out of their will but become the norm sooner or later.

Kiss up, Kick down

Have you heard of this situation before? You probably haven't heard the name but should be familiar with the experience. It is a term used to describe a situation where employees placed somewhere in the middle of the hierarchy of an organization are somewhat polite to those above them but means and abusive to those below them or even their colleagues on the same level!

Everyone ought to be treated equally, but these guys don't care. They exhibit what is also known as eye service to find favor in the sight of their bosses.

Gender Inequality

Don't tell me you weren't expecting to see this. I'm not even sure if I can label this work complete if this subject isn't discussed.

We already have a picture painted in our heads when we hear the term Gender Inequality, mainly about men and women not being treated equally due to certain factors like biology, psychology, or cultural norms prevalent in society.

But then, what about the workplace? I've said before that almost everything happens in the workplace. It's like a small society that mirrors the larger community it finds itself in and incorporates nearly everything good or bad into its system.

In 2008, female medical doctors who had just become qualified in New York State had a starting salary of $16,819 less than their male counterparts. That speaks volumes. Then come to think of what it entails for women who are black. Then we'd be merging the racial and gender factors, and that wouldn't be too nice a combination, would it? I'm afraid no. But it's the reality anyway. As in society, people are valued in the workplace by their gender, with the female gender usually being on the losing end. Despite whatever qualifications she may have or expertise she may exhibit.

Employers sometimes don't care about the potential they might miss out on to satisfy their conscience, which is wrong. If you ask me, whatever strategy a business owner may come up with, no matter how good that strategy is at ensuring growth and stability in the enterprise, if an all-embracing system isn't in play, that strategy may not achieve its full potential. People either fail to see this or see it and still ignore it.

The Toxic Workplace

I want to describe the toxic workplace as the result of the above factors and much more. It is like the term which encompasses all forms of ills in the workplace. Sometimes, not only employers or superiors who make up the toxic workplace. Employees play their roles as well in making the workplace unconducive for others. Sometimes these employees are even more trouble than their bosses and cause problems for them!

A "toxic workplace" refers to an office environment characterized by significant personal conflicts between coworkers whose actions can harm the overall productivity of whatever firm they work for. A toxic workplace is often seen as the result of poisonous employers and toxic employees who are motivated by their desire for personal gain (power, money, fame, or special status), using unethical means to manipulate and get on the nerves of those around them psychologically; the motives are to grow or increase power, money or special status or divert attention away from their awful performance and misdeeds at work.

These people exercise little or no care about the duty they owe the organization for which they work or their co-workers in terms of ethics or professional conduct toward others. They define relationships with co-workers not by organizational structure but by co-workers they favor and those they do not like or trust.

Working in a place alongside these kinds of people can toy with your feelings a lot. Even when you're not a direct victim of their toxicity, just seeing them display their toxic traits daily at work can sometimes be tiring or even traumatic.

Just imagine watching a dedicated co-worker who probably works harder than everyone else in the office being mistreated, underpaid, slandered, and the likes because of her skin color or because she didn't say yes to the sexual demands of her boss. That can do a lot of psychologically damaging things to anyone who has a conscience. Then what if, just what if you were a direct victim of such toxicity in the workplace?

It would help if you were on the lookout for sure signs in trying to identify toxic workplaces. If you're not already aware of them, I'm here to help, always! You should know that you can count on me anytime, any day! Here are a few signs that you notice in a toxic workplace;

Fatigue and Ill Health

Toxic workplaces will often make you feel stressed out, tired, and ill due to the level of stress you may be trying to endure. So, if you find yourself calling in sick often or constantly feeling drained and exhausted, it may indicate that your work environment is negatively affecting your health.

Lack of Enthusiasm

While at work, scan your office or work area well and search for signs of genuine happiness. It can equal toxicity if you're unable to notice positive conversations or employees socializing. This lack of motivation can rub off on everyone in the workspace, creating a more significant problem.

Low Turnover Rate

If you begin to observe a low turnover rate at your company or your workspace, it may point out that other workers have picked up on the toxic vibe in the workplace. Poor morale, sickness, and an overall lack of enthusiasm will certainly lead employees to seek employment opportunities elsewhere.

Stifled Growth

If your organization doesn't offer learning opportunities or mentorship, I'm afraid they may not be invested in your growth. Of course, it may not be the company's responsibility to motivate you to continue learning and improve yourself, but the lack of support can indicate a toxic workplace. They're only interested in taking from you but not adding to you. That's toxic enough.

COPING WITH WORKPLACE TOXICITY

While we have learned a few signs to note if your workplace is toxic, it's also essential to know how to handle these struggles if you do not plan to quit anytime soon. To me, leaving is always an option. It only depends on how long a person is willing to endure or when such a person finds an alternative.

We should also have in mind the fact that what works for others may not work for you. So do well to figure out what works for you, and don't kill yourself trying to fit in a particular style.

Having said quite enough, here are a few ways to deal with a toxic work environment.

Find Support

Support comes in handy in any situation, toxic workplace; it's essential to have people who stay by you no matter what position you find yourself in. You should see this support outside your place of work rather than in your workplace. Because while you may feel uncomfortable venting to your colleagues at work, your support system outside work allows you an outlet to express your emotions and frustrations without reservations.

Stay Positive

Spending so much time around toxic people can negatively affect your mood. Staying positive should be your priority, even if you don't find yourself around uplifting personalities, to keep you from never-ending negativity. Always remind yourself of the good part about your job and look for the good in as much as you can. When you're always focused on what you're grateful for, you're not going to allow the negativity to get to you.

Also, remember that seeing the good in something is not equal to being utterly blind to what you're not comfortable with.

Take a Break

There should always be time to step away from your duties. Taking a short break gives your brain time to rest. Take walks, meditate or eat a healthy snack. Just try as much as possible to leave your workspace for a short period as it can improve your mood and overall productivity when you return to work.

Meditate

Take a few minutes out of your work break to meditate as it helps to cultivate peace and calm in your mind. Take deep breaths in a rhythmic pattern, focusing on every breath you take and relieving any tension and stress.

Surround Yourself With Positivity

There are different kinds of personalities you find in the workplace. It's for your good that you hang around the positive ones. Having them around can help you survive toxicity. Make it a goal to spend as much time as possible with them. You are providing support for them and socializing with them throughout the day.

Quit

If you can't take it anymore, it's OK to admit that you can't. Don't force things. But before you leave, make sure you have some other opportunities and that you're a hundred percent sure of the decision.

AFFIRMATIONS

1. I am a masterpiece, and I am good at what I do.
2. Amidst toxicity, my self-worth remains intact.
3. I will not be a reflection of a toxic workplace
4. I am in control of my actions and responsible for the consequences
5. I have no room for negativity
6. I will not be a contributing factor to a toxic work environment
7. I am a smart and intelligent black woman
8. There's always an option for me; I will always have a choice
9. I refuse to be objectified by anyone, whoever they might be
10. I will always see the good in everything
11. I am not a moron; I will not be blind to my struggles
12. I am not a party to gossip and small talk.
13. I am the boss of my life
14. I am a pillar of support to others.
15. I am surrounded by positivity
16. I am not stagnant; I crave growth.
17. There's always a reason to be grateful
18. I have a bright future
19. I radiate good energy amid the toxicity
20. I will always be productive and wise with my time because there's a lot to achieve
21. I strive to be consistent at work
22. I choose to remain positive because success begins with the mindset
23. I am letting go of what I can't control to focus on the things I can
24. I will not always feel my best every day, and that's fine.
25. I will make mistakes along the way, and that's fine and normal
26. I will not make rest a luxury but a priority for me

27. Where I work and what I work as don't define my worth
28. I will always make time for family and friends no matter the schedule
29. Even when it gets hard to do, I treat every co-worker with respect
30. I will not allow anyone to take me off course on any day at work
31. I will remain calm when dealing with difficult people
32. When I need to be, I will be honest with my colleagues and will not be offended when they are with me.
33. I will always be confident when sharing my ideas and talent
34. I can go after whatever I want; I have given myself that permission.
35. I embody excellence.

KEY POINTS

1. Society and all its components reflect in every workplace
2. There should always be a limit to endurance
3. Psychological stress always has a way of affecting you physically
4. Find support and surround yourself with positivity always
5. Adopt practices to cope with toxicity while searching for a better place
6. Always know when to quit.

CHAPTER FIVE

FRIENDSHIPS

"Remember that the most valuable antiques are dear old friends".
-H. Jackson Brown, Jr.

We had to get to this point, ladies; it is essential to get to this discussion because if we're talking about life, we've got to talk about friendship. If we're going to be talking about how to improve lives, one of the focal points for discussion has to be FRIENDSHIPS.

In my own opinion, I think this aspect of human life is not given the needed attention. What's more? The word is even misused; it is misunderstood most of the time! It has been treated so casually that people no longer know the true meaning of friendship. And that is why they use it to describe almost every relationship.

But the truth remains that there are words for specific situations. You don't have to call it friendship, your colleague at the desk opposite you, doesn't have to be your friend, the guy or the girl you share a desk with at school doesn't have to be your friend, even your roommate doesn't have to be called a friend! What other scenarios are there? Just name it. Many people misunderstand the concept of friendship and become surprised when people expect to turn up for them in certain situations because they called friends to fail to do so. No girl! She's not a bad friend, she was just never a friend, and that's not her fault!

Why not define relationships properly and stop taking things as you feel or think they are instead of taking things as they are?

There's so much to discuss on the subject, and we'll approach it to step by step. Let us know what friendship is, stop forcing relationships, and improve our lives!

WHAT ARE FRIENDSHIPS?

Friendships can be defined as relationships of affection that exist mutually between people, a more vital form of interpersonal relationship than an "acquaintance" or an "association," such as a classmate, coworker, neighbor, or colleague. Like I said earlier, we should not be too quick to qualify these other relationships as friendships because, most of the time, they do not turn out to be so.

A person may realize he has developed a strong bond with another person over the years without even knowing it. That's where the term "best friend" comes in. Many people in today's world want to choose that kind of friendship. But to me, that kind of friendship chooses you both! It is not a conscious effort; it just happens consistently and will take a while before any of the parties eventually realizes that Oh! This guy's been my buddy for so many years; how did I not know? Yeah, you didn't know because that's how it's supposed to be; you don't force it.

Different people have established various definitions of friendship, and I will talk about them. But it amazes me to see so many rules, theories, and the sort, bordering around something that I feel should be natural!

For instance, many people say "three is a crowd," and therefore, three people cannot be best friends or close friends. They even go as far as drawing conclusions on trios and telling them it'll never work because the world says "three is a crowd." They have specific reasons to back their claims, which may be valid, but I still have many questions!

Friendship results from human emotions, what people feel for each other, which hardly anyone but themselves could decipher. So I wonder how people can make these condescending theories about friendship and want to quickly draw lines or plant red flags on a certain kind of friendship.

Most of the time, a trio may not turn out well and doesn't make a trio a friendly one to run away from when it comes naturally. There are friend groups of 5 to 7 that flourish for years and would probably be the same for long, so what's all these fusses about friendship and the metrics brought about by different scholars or whatever they might be?
In my opinion, it all comes down to you, girl. How do you feel about the friendship? That's all that matters and nothing else! You have to put yourself and your feelings over that of the psychologists who are entitled to their opinion too, but those opinions don't have to be a standard for your friendship. If you're in a trio and it makes you feel good, loved, and cared for, choose that over what anyone has to say because it is a personal issue, and the opinion of others doesn't matter much.

FORMS OF FRIENDSHIPS

This is an aspect of this subject that so many people have had so many different takes on. I'll tell you the simple fact; inconsistency is annoying because when a concept has too many opinions about it, it may lose its authenticity, and the real meaning will be lost along with it. Why not? So many people have a lot to say, and a good percentage of them may be wrong and misleading, unfortunately.

Be careful not to miss the point and make the best of whatever works for you because that matters the most.

For this part, I'd like to toe the path of the great Greek philosopher Aristotle. He says that there are only three kinds of friendship. And I love the distinction. It reflects what happens in our reality today—an absolute truth.

So What Does He Say?

According to the Macedonian-born Greek philosopher, the three kinds of friendships that exists are:

- Friendships of Utility
- Friendships of Pleasure
- Friendships of the Good

These three kinds of friendships will be explored below for a better understanding.

Friendships Of Utility

These kinds of friendships exist between two people who have found out that they will consistently be of benefit to each other. It exists between you and someone who will be helpful to you somehow and vice-versa. Without those benefits, the purpose of such friendship will be defeated.

For example, you've got a co-worker, preferably working at the next desk, which helps you work on stuff when they're too much for you to handle. You help cover for him when he's out somewhere else for a different engagement, you know, stuff like that, and it goes both ways, consistently, not one doing more than the other. That is what Aristotle regards as a friendship of utility.

More like an *"I scratch your back, you scratch mine"* kind of relationship between two people.

I once had a friend during the COVID-19 pandemic, where we all had to work remotely. He was always there to call me for impromptu meetings we had when I happened to be offline, and I would also do the same. On the day he couldn't be online to attend meetings, I would cover up for him; on the days I couldn't be online to participate in discussions, he would do the same.

We had small talks about the duty we had placed on ourselves, but we were both aware of what we suddenly became close to and had unconsciously set limits that we didn't venture beyond. With the pandemic being over, we didn't have much need for each other anymore, and though we tried to start something when we both saw each other's life, the spark wasn't present anymore. The use we both had for each other was no longer present, so sooner or later, we had become like strangers again.

It shouldn't be surprising how we both "fell off" if you want to go out that way. A need brought us together. We both had something to benefit from each other, and that's why we became close in the first place. And with that thing not being in existence anymore, there was no need for friendship anymore, so even if we tried to breed something after the market was gone, it might not have worked because there was no need for the company anymore. We understood that and accepted it the way it was. One critical thing I want you to note about this story is that we understood what we both had back then during the pandemic and realized that we couldn't have that chemistry anymore since there was no spark to it. So we both did not complain that we were slowly drifting apart because we both knew what we became friends for, and it had ended. So what's the need for any charade? We both continued living like nothing ever happened between us during the pandemic.

It's that simple how this kind of friendship works when there's understanding. Any company would work when there is a mutual understanding between both parties about precisely what friendship both have.

Now, I am dropping a hint on how big of a role understanding plays in friendship. Let's move on.

Friendship of Pleasure

Well, as the title connotes, this friendship exists between two people who tend to enjoy the company of each other. The most common scenario is when you want such a person because they are a funny person or are willing to do something to make you feel good. Maybe they have a video game you can play during your free time and be on the same football team or whatever sport you both enjoy.

It's a mutual relationship, so you would also have something to offer to such a person to make that person want to be in your company.

A question, however, could arise as to where the "Friends with Benefit" card would come into play. Whether in the first category or this one. The reason is that, with regards to the first type, you could use each other for sexual satisfaction, and with the second type, you could like each other because of how you make yourselves feel in bed.

I feel the connection between the second kind of friendship would be more robust. This is because, according to the great Aristotle, for the company of pleasure, we would like more than one aspect of the friends we tend to keep for fun. Apart from the sexual satisfaction, one party provides, one might also like his wit, her compassion, or his flirty manner, for instance. On the other hand, friendships of utility exist mainly because the person can help us somehow. And without both parties providing almost the same assistance, that friendship would not work as it is meant to.

Friendships Of The Good

These kinds of friendships have their foundation in mutual respect and admiration. These friendships take much longer to build than the other two types discussed above, and as a result, they're also more powerful and enduring.

These kinds of friendships often materialize when both parties recognize that they have similar values, goals, and ambitions, have similar visions for how the world (or at least their lives) should be, and both work towards achieving what they plan on achieving, Not infrequently. More often than

not, this kind of friendship begins in childhood, adolescence, or college, even if plenty still forms after that, too.
These kinds of friendships are primarily unconditional.

They're not there because you have a use for them; you're not here because they take pleasure in being around you; they're there just because you're you and because they mean a lot to you. Such a friend doesn't have to do a thousand and one thing for the other party to kindle the friendship, nor have to do whatever the other party enjoys gaining this friendship. This friendship is purely genuine, and there are no strings attached.

This friendship encompasses all other companies and should be the standard for a true friendship.
This is what I regard as friendship in the first place. Because I value friendship so much, any other relationship named "friendship" doesn't portray what friendship truly is, is not and will never be friends to me.

According to Aristotle, whom I agree with, the third kind of friendship is the most important among the three types of friendships. These are friendships founded on mutual respect for one another, appreciation for each other's qualities, and a solid will to assist others in need because they believe in each other and recognize their greatness. To me, this is the only relationship that should be termed friendship.

The first two types of friendship can be broken or lost easily. The driving force behind those kinds of relationships is one's utility and pleasure. These friendships will probably fade off when benefits are achieved or a change of common interest. However, companies based on goodness are usually long-lasting.

And people that'll value your friendship, not because of what you have to offer or what they stand to gain from you, but for genuine reasons, are hard to find and develop, and If you happen to have more than a handful of friends based on goodness, you are indeed blessed. My mother always says, *"Friends will tell you what you desire to hear, buts good friends tell you what you need to hear."*

Having looked at the three kinds of friendships Aristotle spoke about, how about we talk about the company's qualities?

The subject is broad, and if anyone plans to cover everything up on friendship, such a person would have to write a full-fledged book.

So let's move on to our next subject for discussion.
QUALITIES OF A FRIEND

It is vital to note that when it comes to friendship, you must never choose quantity over quality. That's like a taboo. Having ten people you call your friends, or you think you are your friends when they're not, is much worse than having three genuine people who know the value and worth of friendship.

The following are some of the qualities you would want to look out for when breeding friendships with other people;

Loyalty

Do you have a friend who forsakes everything to help you at the point of your need? That is someone whom you can call a friend and not a person you should play with. Hold them tight and close because their type is rare. Always being there when we need them the most, helping to lighten our burden, providing a shoulder to lean on, and also helping to shoulder the inevitable hurdles, stresses, and crises that life throws at us. They can transform what seems to be an unfathomable mountain into a small hill that can be easily accessed. They are always there to make things easy.

You shouldn't trade such a person for anything in the world because it won't be easy getting such a person ever again.

Trust Worthiness

No friendship should leave trust out of the list. That box must be ticked! Every relationship needs trust as its bedrock and foundation to stand firm. Friendship is not an exception when every relationship is mentioned. Therefore, one of the qualities of a good friend is that they are trustworthy and genuine.

Do not be ashamed to tell someone you call a friend about your weaknesses, imperfections, or shortcomings. You should trust them enough to keep it a secret when you tell them to, and if you don't, you should reconsider your friendship with such a person.

Acceptance

A friend will accept you for all your perfections and imperfections. And you're not going to feel uneasy being in their company because they have made you feel safe and comfortable, irrespective of your shortcomings.

Even though you are not in any way perfect hence, you can be yourself around them. That's one of the pleasures a good friendship allows you to enjoy. You can afford to be yourself around them because they have acknowledged and accepted that not everyone can be perfect, and you happen to be among them. A good friend will get you despite your flaws and love you wholly.

Listening Ears

No one doesn't need someone to listen to them actively. Imagine being in a situation where you need your friend to listen and pay attention to what you have to say, but they do the exact opposite. It would, in many ways, make you sad, wouldn't it?

And then a friend who always lends a listening ear to what you have to say engages with you and even offers a solution to any problem you may have been experiencing. Isn't that blissful? It sure is!

Reciprocity

There are a lot of qualities to be considered when building friendship, but I may have to draw the curtains here. And there's no better quality to conclude with than this.

We must understand that in everything we do with other people, striking a balance in any relationship is essential, especially the one of giving and taking. The quality of a good friendship is that reciprocity exists, no one should be selfish about most of their needs, and this will lead to a relationship where both parties will be satisfied.

This does not mean that one friend carries all the burden in the relationship; it means that, while one has the ball, the other does too. When the support comes from just one side of the relationship, the supporter will give up at some point.

Some friends would outdo the other, but this is fine so long as the other party reciprocates the gesture because some people are naturally born to give more.
To me, the purpose of friendship will be defeated without reciprocity.

Why do I have to lend anyone a listening ear when they won't do the same for me?
What's the need to accept a person when they will not accept you?
Why would anyone want to be loyal to someone else if that person will not return the energy?

These are not selfish questions but reasonable questions that need to be adequately answered before one ventures into any friendship that will most likely not bring satisfaction.

It's that simple. If you can't return the energy, then there's no need to give you in the first place.

To conclude, all these qualities you wish to see in other people, you should see first in yourself. Aside from finding and being with a good friend, you have to be a good friend so that compatibility can exist. If you're not willing to be a good friend to a person, then there's no need to make friends with such a person, and that's on, period!

AFFIRMATIONS

1. I am a great friend
2. I can tell my friend anything I want to
3. I attract amazing friends to my life
4. I am not ashamed of being myself around my friends
5. My friends are one of the sources of happiness in my life
6. let go of toxic relationships with ease
7. I reciprocate in the best way I can
8. I can rely on my friends always
9. I have deep connections with my friends.
10. New people come into my life at the right time
11. I will always offer support to my friends
12. I will always lend a listening ear to anything they have to say.
13. When I can, I'll always be there for my friends.
14. I will attract the perfect friends when I'm ready to make new friends.
15. Every day, I attract positive and amazing people.
16. I will not run after people who will let me down.
17. I'm imperfect; my friends are, too; it doesn't get to me.
18. I always feel safe around my friends as they feel around me.
19. I make friends that I genuinely admire
20. All my friends and beautiful in their unique way
21. I will always make sure to set healthy boundaries
22. I constantly let my friends know how much they mean to me
23. I will always be able to talk to my friends about something
24. I can say no to my friends, and they'll understand
25. My friends do not judge me, and I also do not consider them
26. I can always make new friends when I lose the old ones
27. I genuinely want the best for my friends, and they want the same as well

28. I attract friendships that bring me joy
29. No matter how long a company lasts, it'll always add value to my life
30. I can walk away from friendships that cause me pain
31. I will always value positive relationships.
32. I attract healthy and worthy friendships.
33. I forgive myself for all the times I stayed in toxic friendships.
34. I do not attract friendships that trouble my soul.
35. I attract friendships that align with my goals in life.
36. I am not afraid to move away from friendships that make me less of myself.

KEY POINTS

1. Friendships happen naturally.
2. Everyone has to play their part in a friendship
3. One must be willing to sacrifice in friendships
4. Friends ought to learn how to accept each other's weaknesses
5. A friend in need is a friend indeed.

CHAPTER SIX

FINANCES

"I believe that through knowledge and discipline, financial peace is possible for all of us."
-Dave Ramsey

We all think of one thing when we hear "Finance." Do I need to tell you? Money, of course!

Money? Who on earth doesn't take money seriously? I'm yet to find anyone who doesn't, honestly. That's to show you how much importance money holds in the world today.

But to tell you the truth, the word finances holds much more than money. Of course, money is part of it, but there's a lot to finance beyond just having money at your disposal. And we're going to be looking at what's more.

Finance studies the discipline of money, currency, and capital assets. It is related to but isn't the same as economics, which is the study of production, distribution, and consumption of money, assets, goods, and services. I don't want to sound too educational, so it has to be broken down into bits where we can deal with our concerns about finances because it is a vast topic.

There are mainly three areas of finance generally.

We have Personal Finances, defined as "the mindful planning of monetary spending and saving, while also having in mind the possibility of future risk." Personal finance usually involves:

- Paying for education.
- Financing durable goods such as real estate and cars.
- Buying insurance.
- Investing.
- Saving for retirement.

The major areas of personal finance are income, spending, saving, investing, and protection.

Then we have Corporate Finances, which deals with the actions that managers take to increase the firm's worth to the shareholders, the sources of funding and the capital structure of corporations, and the tools and analysis involved in the allocation of financial resources. So this is finances catering for a business or a corporation.

And then lastly, we have the public finances, which describes finance as related to sovereign states, sub-national entities, and associated public entities or agencies, which means finances relating to nations or states.

With all that has been said so far, it should be pretty clear what aspect of finances we're about to discuss. Not that the others don't affect our daily lives in specific ways, they do. But we will deal with aspects closer to our personal lives and finances.

With money being a necessity in today's world, it has become essential to know how to spend when we earn.

And this is not restricted to a particular class of people. Everybody needs to learn the art of money, whether you make a million dollars a month or just a thousand. Everyone needs to know the workings of money and how to manage it. Because failing to do so, will undoubtedly bring about waste and other unforeseen costs that may accrue to money mismanagement.

So, here we go! The big topic!

PERSONAL FINANCES

Concerning personal finance, the term is mainly used to describe the financial management of a person or a family's resources. It is made up of how one manages their money through expenses, investments, and savings, taking into consideration various unforeseen life events and risks.

Other personal finance aspects include banking, budgeting, retirement, insurance, estate planning, and more.

The term stands for the entire financial industry in a person's life, which encompasses all the bodies that offer financial services to an individual.

The main focus of personal finances is on meeting the financial goals of an individual or a person, both long and short term. Whether you have enough money for your monthly bills or want to plan for your retirement, it all depends on how well you can sort out your finances.

Suppose one has attained a certain level of financial literacy. In that case, it plays a massive role in helping such a person to know the difference between financial decisions that will be beneficial and that which will be detrimental to their financial future.

Having a plan for your finances will help you meet your short- and long-term needs without exceeding your income limits.

The truth is, it's better to start planning your finances sooner than later. So, you shouldn't be left out in this race, my beautiful young black lady. You have to take steps to improve the quality of your life, and this is one of them. So I urge you to follow through, as there are many things to be learned here.

The Essence of Personal Finances

There are specific reasons why knowing about our finances is important. A few out of many will be treated below;

Meeting Money Needs

Everyone has to understand this simple truth. Money issues are beyond what most of us know. We must look at the bigger picture when we approach this subject. This way, we can think beyond just going to work and making money at the end of the month or however we get paid.

You should be able to ask yourself,

"What comes after making that money? Do we spend?" Well, this shouldn't be the case.

When we ask ourselves these questions, our answers are supposed to help us draw out plans that establish how much our income is, what our expenses are, what plans we may have, as well as our future financial objectives. That is how you think beyond just working to earn money because that's not all there is to life.

Managing Your Income

If one fails to plan for their income, they will either overspend or spend on unnecessary items. Still, with a proper financial plan, one can manage theirs effectively.

Planning will enable you to spend your money on what is necessary and save or invest the rest.

Furthermore, managing your income will help you draw out a priority list, giving you an idea of the expenses to take care of. You can also effectively know how much is necessary for tax payments, savings, or clearing your monthly bills. Ain't that cool?

Budgeting, Spending, Saving, and Investing

Financial stability doesn't wholly depend on having a fat paycheck at the end of the month. That is one butter truth most people don't want to accept. A person who earns a $500,000 salary every month can still be living in a substantial financial crisis if they fail to plan for that income. It is because they may be spending much more than they are earning, sometimes without knowing about it.

On the contrary, a person earning less than 500k a month could still live a more financially stable life than the former. It will be so if such a person has drawn out a suitable plan for his income, saves, and lives within his means. It's that simple.

Good personal finance skills help you to understand how much you earn, what your monthly expenses are, and how you can budget within that income.

Many people may regard it as living stingy. Still, I call it sticking to what your budget indicates, and it does a great deal in helping one avoid so many overspending temptations that they otherwise would have ignored.
For example, you will be able to resist the temptation of purchasing a luxury gadget to fit in a friends club by looking at your budget and checking if that can fit into your list.

If your income doesn't allow it, or you have some other things planned, you can forgo the shifting. You can achieve this if you have a budget and stick to it diligently. If you don't have a budget drawn, I'm afraid you will have nothing to stick to and end up overspending and having a lot of regrets later on.

As Dave Ramsey said, *"Don't spend more than you earn!" This is a simple rule you must adhere to live a financially comfortable life."*

Having the Family Financially Secured

Somewhere near the top of every woman's priority list is financial security for them and their families. Everyone wants to be assured that they can cater to the money needs of their family, in a failing economy or not.

It even hurts to think of their families suffering due to a lack of money, especially when they are not around to help. It is the most common reason people struggle to earn enough money that can offer them a sense of security for years to come.

Many people fail to realize that the answer does not lie entirely in how much one earns but also in how much income is planned. The truth is, if you want to have financial freedom and security, you must learn to make sound financial plans.

Lastly, with healthy insurance policies and investments, you and your family won't suffer financially.

Keeping Off Bad Debts

Having little debts is not much of a problem. But being overly in debt is where the problem lies and can be very dangerous to your future finances. It's necessary to be able to manage one's obligations in such a way that guarantees that no damage is done to your future financial stability.

Wanting to grow your wealth quickly is equivalent to knowing how to manage your debts, which is why personal finance is critical to ensure this happens.

One way to stay off debt is to avoid overspending or spending more than you earn.

Improving the Standard of Living

One vital importance of financial planning is helping you improve your living standards. But how can personal finance help you achieve this feat?

The truth is that the more you plan for your finances, the more your savings will be. This means that instead of more money going to unplanned expenses, more will be saved. Higher savings will enable you to manage during financially challenging times.

To conclude, I must say.

Studying your finances is one big step to having a stable financial future. Very few are aware of this.
And although some will not realize early enough to make a change until they are too deep in a financial crisis, I can only

hope that my beautiful black ladies wouldn't disappoint me and be one of those who will always ask, "why is personal finance important?" after this discussion, change for the better now, and impact your future finances before it's too late.

RULES OF PERSONAL FINANCE

Having spoken about the need for personal finance for our young black women who will change the world, some rules ought to be followed to the teeth if possible to ensure that our finances wouldn't be in chaos at the end of the day.

Let's peruse the rules together, and you'll promise me you'll practice them. I believe you can! Because a black woman can do anything, she is determined to do to make her life better, and I can't help but be elated being able to play my part in all these. Yay! I'm pumped! Let's go!

Have a Goal

If you have no defined goals, it won't be easy to know what personal financial success entails. Define your destination, and then create a realistic step-by-step plan that helps you achieve them.

Start Saving Early

Time has a way of being against us and can also be our best friend. When saving, time is going to be your best friend when you start saving early enough, say in your early 20s. And not only will you have more time to build wealth (even on a modest salary), but you'll also have more time for compounding interest to work its magic.

Distinguish Wants From Needs

People find it hard to separate their wants from their needs. It may sound absurd, but these are issues, and it only leaves them in a constant state of financial unrest. But I want you to understand that human needs are pretty simple — food, clothing, shelter, health care, reliable transportation, etc. To me, everything else is a want. But that doesn't mean we shouldn't indulge in desires from time to time (life would be boring if we couldn't). It is what I'm trying to tell you. Choose your wants consciously, and do not let their constant pursuit jeopardize your financial security. It's not going to be worth it at the end of the day, trust me.

Differentiate between Assets and Liabilities

Just in case you're having a hard time drawing a line of distinction, here's a simple definition: Assets are valuable things that belong to you. Your car, house, and savings account are assets. Liabilities are simply debts. Student loans are an example. Now that you've known the difference, I'm trying to convey the message that you should try your best to accumulate assets and reduce liabilities.

Live Within Your Means

Drawing up a solid budget (one that you must stick to) and not living above gives you automatic freedom from the frustrating cycle of working, overspending, servicing debt, and working some more—such a hard way to live a life, I guess. But you can make life easy by learning to live within your means.

Do you know what's better? Living below your means. This is because spending less than you earn leaves you with a surplus — the vital capital that funds your future. It works like magic; you have to try it, ladies; you have to!

Don't Invest in Anything You Don't Understand

For anyone to succeed in an investing venture, it will take critical thinking, discipline, and consistency over time. It is not advisable to take shortcuts, and investing in overly complex products you don't understand will most likely cause a big blow to your long-term gains and capital. Stick with what you know, young woman; a lot is happening in the financial markets now, from Crypto to NFTs and a lot more. If you're yet to understand those, there's no need to invest in them. Don't be carried away by the crowd; most people don't know what they're doing, and you black woman must be different from them. If you're interested, you must learn extensively about them before investing your money in such ventures. Strive to learn more every day, and don't be spooked by cyclical fluctuations in the market.

Settle Debts With the Highest Interest Rate First

If you cannot avoid consumer debt, you've got to apply strategic wisdom in how you pay it off. Simply paying off high-interest balances first exposes you to fewer interest charges over time.

Prepare for Emergencies

Stack up to six to eight months' net income in an emergency fund. It's a simple but effective way to cushion the effects of unforeseen circumstances like a reduction, poor health, unexpected household expenses, and other life events that could threaten your family's purse.

And then, to wrap things up, you must remember that in making preparations for the unexpected, you also have to include proper estate planning. Guarding your assets and providing for your family is often ignored as a golden rule of smart personal finance. If you're yet to make a will, add it to your to-do list and make sure to do that!

Educate Yourself

It'll be reasonable to conclude this segment with this information, wouldn't it? I guess so. You see, many personal finance books are out in the open. I wish this stuff were taught in every high school and college, but it isn't, unfortunately. So you have to prepare yourself. Besides, no one will care more about your money decisions than you. Invest in yourself! It's the best investment you can make. In the long run, the benefits will materialize if you're severe enough.

Oh, beautiful women! I wish I could go on and on because I enjoy the ride. But the coach's going to have to stop here.

I want to let you know that you're capable of achieving anything you set your mind to because you're strong, and your energy never runs out.

I admire your courage and will to outdo yourselves every time. That makes you a black woman, ready to defy all odds and become who you want to be.

I will support you all the way; even if it means me staying up all night typing these words of encouragement, I'm ready to do that to let you know how special you are to me and the world at large.

The world is waiting for your glow! Go on and be Champions, and I'll be at the corner applauding your prowess, smiling like a proud coach.

Go on and win, ladies!

AFFIRMATIONS

1. New income opportunities will come to me
2. My finances will blossom
3. I can rely on my judgments to make sound financial choices.
4. I am wealthy beyond money.
5. My life is rich and full.
6. I will achieve my financial goals.
7. I can change the world for the better with my money
8. I am allowed to be successful and be happy
9. I'm going to use my money to do good to myself and the people I love
10. I can be comfortable with cash when I manage it well.
11. I am smart with my money.
12. It's enjoyable to spend responsibly.
13. I'm capable of saving money to ensure my financial freedom.
14. I won't be a hindrance to leading a financially secure life.
15. I believe in myself making intelligent financial decisions.
16. I can overcome my spending impulses.
17. Spending money responsibly makes me happy
18. I deserve and expect financial freedom

19. I am capable of building and completing a financial foundation.
20. I receive financial success.
21. My finances don't scare me; I have a plan
22. I can always find the positives in my money issues
23. My income can exceed my expenses
24. Hard work will bring me money
25. I can have fun in a frugal way
26. I will be grateful to myself in the future for saving money
27. It gives me joy when I spend money wisely
28. I spend money on what matters to me
29. I enjoy saving my money
30. Generational wealth is always a possibility and within reach.
31. I lead a financially stable life.
32. Wealth knows me by name.
33. I forgive myself for all the times I worked against my financial stability.
34. I embrace wealth for myself and my generation.
35. I am worthy of a high income.
36. I have all it takes to earn the salary I desire.
37. I attract all that I deserve.
38. I do not drown in lack.
39. I am wealthy.
40. I do not accept substandard treatment for my excellence.
41. I love what I do, and I do it well.

KEY POINTS

1. Financial literacy is a crucial step to financial freedom
2. Never live above your means; try as much as possible to live below it.
3. Accumulate assets and let go of liabilities
4. Never stop saving
5. Investing in yourself is the best.

CHAPTER SEVEN

THE CAREER WOMAN

"Every great dream begins with a dreamer. Always remember, you have the strength, the patience, and the passion for reaching for the stars to change the world."
-Harriet Tubman

You probably must have been wondering why I didn't treat this earlier. Do you know why? I'll tell you the truth; I honestly do not understand why as well, ladies. I'll concede.

When I conclude this book, and I, unfortunately, discover that I forgot to add this topic, I'll be mad at myself and make adjustments.

Because a career is something that no woman should neglect, and it's rather sad that many women want to settle for less in their husbands' homes, doing the laundry, the dishes, changing the diapers, you know... and all the other stuff homemakers do. Now I'm not saying that a woman should do these things! That's not my point. My point is that some women want to do these things every day for the rest of their lives!

Not to sound overly ambitious, but you ladies shouldn't have to settle for that! That's straight-up demeaning! And it's what you want? Be honest and don't let life's circumstances define your ambitions; that's your job! So you have to take it on!

It hurts to see women settling for the bare minimum and depending wholly on their partners for support of various kinds. Not to sound rude, but there's no dignity in that for me.

You all are go-getters! Not hiding under the wings of someone else's ambitions! That's unacceptable to me. Or you probably come from a wealthy home and don't see the need to be hardworking because you have everything you want and need on your back and call? Are you kidding me? Don't you know what it took for your parents to get to that point? Or let's assume you don't know and you only heard stories.

But then how about when you become a Mommy? That should hit, I guess.

You may have the money to give them a better life, probably because your parents left a fortune, but how will they look up to you? What are they going to see in their mommy that will inspire them?

This is why this topic is important! Any form of mediocrity shouldn't be tolerated in your space. You can be whatever you want, black beauty, your skin emulates toughness, and go through whatever you need to get to where you are!

You've got this lady! It would be best if you trusted me by now because we've come a long way together, and I'll need you to do that when I say again that I got your back till the very end.

Now let's start with the momentum we have built. It always feels good to be a source of empowerment to people.

Let's go!

WHAT DOES A CAREER ENTAIL?

There are a lot of ways to put it. But I'd like to have it this way, personally;

It is that path you want to follow for the rest of your life while searching for opportunities to improve and benefit more as time goes by. Now, this is not what you need to do because you need the money or something of that sort; this is what you want to do and excel in!

A career is mainly driven by love and passion for a particular path, and that's why it's pretty different from a job. (We'd treat that as soon as we can as we progress)

For example, one can choose to play football as their career, may not earn immediately from the start, but finds ways to improve themselves while wanting to benefit from it as well. That's a career path. Not one that you immediately gain from for gaining sake, but once you find peace in what you enjoy doing all the time, the word is passion! That's a career.

How about art? We see music, dance, poetry, drawing, painting, and the rest. And then the sciences! Medicine, Engineering, man! There's so much to say, and the list is inexhaustible!

That is what a career path means to me, and nothing has and will change. You should also always remember that it's not about what you're capable of doing; it's about how you feel about doing that thing. That's what matters the most. Do you find peace, enjoy it, and want to improve? So many questions to determine what a career entails. We'll go into details much later about that, but then there's something I need you to be clear about.

Look out.

A JOB AND A CAREER

These words are helpful interchangeably, and it's one of the things that honestly annoy me. Although related, these are two completely different things that shouldn't be used together to mean the same thing. That's an absolute blunder in its entirety!

A job differs from a career by miles on end, and we'll find out why. But let me first define what a job is.

A job can be defined as a duty a person is expected or obliged to do; a piece of work and more like a specific activity which is carried out as part of the routine of one's occupation or for an agreed price which will be paid at the end of an agreed specified time.

So while we ask how a job and a career differ, certain areas should be examined to dissect the distinction.
We're only going to discuss a few, so here we go.

Requirements

The requirements of both concepts can help distinguish between them. There's this form of specialized training and education that a person is required to acquire as he chases his career. And also, there's so much individual energy put into pursuing a job, like having to do a series of personal research to add more knowledge to what you may already naturally have; that's what passion drives you to do.

Want to know better so that you can do better? That's one aspect of chasing a career. Is it a music career you want to pursue? Apart from probably having the natural talent for music, there's still a lot of work to do to be up there where you wish to be. And that's one of the things chasing a career entails.

However, on the other hand, having a job requires less. Since it's not your passion, it's not something you want to go all out. You're okay if you're doing what needs to be done at that point. You're content. Not ruling out that you can also be hardworking in your job, but the hunger to strive for more isn't there. It's the means to an end, so do the bare minimum, and that's all.

Time

Time is crucial in all our dealings in life, and if we're yet to realize that, we have a long way to go.
Chasing a career path is a long-term thing. This is what you want to do for the rest of your life, so even the word "long term" may not be an adequate qualification.

I wish I could use "eternal term," but that would be too extreme.

No one puts so much work into something to stick around for 2 to 3 years and then vanish into thin air. That'll be a complete waste of passion and the resources you used to fuel that passion.

So yeah, while chasing your career, you must aim for longevity. Well, in my opinion, everything is dependent on each other. Your longevity depends on the hard work you put in. Because all things are equal, your output is determined by the input, and when the latter is poor, we can't expect much from the former.

Some people have worked so hard in pursuing their careers that even in death, their legacy remains. That's what I'm talking about when I say longevity. So many people don't even have to die before their legacy is erased, and the online time they're remembered is when they finally give up the ghost, and soon enough, we hear nothing from them ever again.

They're so many people who have achieved this feat. I love Michael Jackson, and I think he is one person whose legacy will remain for quite a long time. You can add to the list if you want, but I guess you know what I mean now.

On the other hand, the timespan for a job shouldn't be one to last long. I don't know if I've said this before, but a job is the means to an end, which means the short term. But it is not always so. So many people have resorted to working at a job all the days of their lives whether they love what they're doing or not.

They want to get by, and that can be hurtful not being able to do what you wish to due to circumstances beyond your control. But is that it? Are you sure you can't take control of what you want to do?

That's a question I'd keep asking.

Income

Lastly, I'm going to talk about income. Your income as a career person goes far beyond money. There are a lot of other benefits accrued to a person when he is a top figure in his career. They include fame, recognition, respect, and legacy; it goes on and on. These are the benefits of having a fantastic job.

On the other hand, jobs do not provide many benefits other than money at the end of the day. Don't get this all wrong; there are massively paying jobs, but you don't get much more than money.

But we must understand, however, that a relationship also exists between these two things. That they're different doesn't mean they don't have some connection. They do.

A person usually has several jobs at their disposal in their career, and it is generally easier to switch jobs in the same field of work that defines one's career.

However, changing careers is more complex and may require the person to start at the bottom of the ladder in the new job. And that is one rare thing to do, I must say. Have multiple passions for multiple careers? Superhuman!

CAREER DEVELOPMENT

Everything worth trying requires development and improvement. The word career doesn't fully exist without the word development added to it.
For as long as a person's career is needed long-term, there must always arise a need for development. If there isn't, you're going to be left behind.

Career development involves a series of activities which is aimed at the overall improvement of a person's career. It usually consists in creating new goals regularly and acquiring the necessary skill set to bring those goals to actualization.

It is directly linked to an individual's growth and satisfaction, which pushes them to acquire the knowledge and skills required for the option or career path they have chosen. In addition, after receiving the desired know-how, he has to put them into practice to achieve the goals and targets he has set for himself.

THE STAGES OF CAREER DEVELOPMENT

The number of career development steps varies according to different writers and thinkers. Some say there are four, some say five, and some say six. Well, I'd stick to five because I think it's good to be in between and whether you realize it or not, you'll always have to go through these steps of career development.

Self-Assessment

This is the first step in career development. I'd say it involves two different situations. First, the individual may consciously assess himself on the kind of career and growth they wish to have; on the other hand, it may happen somewhat unconsciously. That's where we see natural gifts and talents coming into play. People find themselves doing something and find out they're good at it. But one thing that's common between the two is that they're both going to require development. Be it a natural talent or a result of self-assessment. Talent without hard work will not do so much as hard work without talent will.

Career Awareness

The second stage of career development involves exploring the various career paths that align with the self-assessment of the talent you've discovered in the first stage. As I earlier mentioned, there's always more to a career, leaving you with options to pick from, picking the one that suits you best after assessing yourself.

For example, another issue arises after thoroughly assessing yourself and you conclude that you want to become a lawyer.

What aspect of the law am I looking to major in? Criminal Law, Commercial Law, Land Law, the list is inexhaustible, but you have to make sure you look at everything thoroughly so that you don't make a mistake to toe the wrong path that may likely land you somewhere you'd regret.

Goal-Setting

I'd say this is a very crucial stage in career development. The most important event is the stage where one clearly defines short-term and long-term goals for actualizing the career one aspires to. Both short-term and long-term goals need to be limited to start with.

Short-term goals need to be done as quickly as possible, while long-term goals can be tweaked and changed as time goes by.

Skill Training

After serving the career and the goals, one needs to acquire the right skills to ensure growth materializes. This can either take personal training or join a structured training program online or offline. These skills have to be acquired to prevent mediocrity as it is the least expected of a career chaser. Once the right skills are developed, one can begin the final stage.

Performing

This is the last stage of career development; the actual performance. After gaining all the proper knowledge and the necessary skills, the critical part is to carry out the tasks and jobs in the career success to grow in the career path.

You need to understand that the five stages of career development do not necessarily need to be followed in the order in which they have appeared here. They're all part of an ongoing process, and even when one has gotten to the last stage, they will always need to revisit the previous steps to get the proper career growth.

These stages are mostly followed unconsciously by people, and that's not supposed to be an issue. As long as career growth is taking place, everything is in place.

FACTORS INFLUENCING CAREER DEVELOPMENT

Career development is affected by several factors and the way they interact with each other. These factors need to be studied to know what career would suit you and what job will not.

Let's have a look.

Personal Characteristics

Your type of personality, interests, and values (especially work-related) all have a role to play in one's career development. Close attention must be paid to these traits while choosing a career because these traits hardly ever leave, and once a mistake is made, it becomes tough to cope. A thorough self-assessment will, however, help you learn about your characteristics and then allow you to find careers that are just the perfect match for you.

Physical and Mental Abilities

It is obvious that some people are a better fit for some careers than others, and this is because of their physical and mental abilities and limitations. Don't you ever overlook the importance of finding an occupation that will make the best use possible of your abilities?

Socio-Economic Factors

Socio-economic factors can be a hindrance to the development of one's career. For example, your financial circumstances may threaten to keep you from attending college, which may be necessary to pursue a particular job you have chosen. On the brighter side, several ways have been dedicated to overcoming these barriers, such as limited financial resources, namely student loans, financial aid, and scholarships.

Chance Factors

These are life events that we have little or no control over. These events can play a significant role in influencing the careers that we choose and how we progress in them. An example could be the need to support a family which is financially keeping you from pursuing an advanced education to develop your career further. You don't have to blame yourself for issues of this manner because they're beyond your control, and there's no need to worry about something beyond your control because there is nothing you can do about it.

IMPROVING YOUR CAREER DEVELOPMENT

The world is evolving, and the evolution is massive and rapid, and you cannot afford to be on the wrong side of everything because you will be left behind, definitely and by miles as well, if you don't want to evolve with it.

Whatever career you find yourself in, you must always find ways to improve to ensure you are always on top of your game. Having enough passion for driving you crazy and craving more would be best.

I have some of these tips for improvement that I'd love to share with you all, and I'm pretty positive they'll be of help.

Here they are;

Learn Everyday

There is getting better at what we already know, and then there's learning new stuff. But whatever the case may be, make sure you understand every day. Learning may come as a challenge; for example, if you're working on a project and you come across some new information that may be vital to your project but you have little or no knowledge about, rather than chicken out, accept the challenge and strive to know more about it. You never know when you will need that piece of information again.

Be Indispensable

You have to strive to be someone they can't do without. Your value increases when you have complete control over what you can do in the career path that you have chosen. You can achieve this through challenging yourself, learning about new things every day, becoming well-grounded in what you already know, and that entire sort. It will help you stand out from the crowd and be invaluable wherever you find yourself.

Interaction

There should always be a need to engage with people on the same career path, primarily those far above you. Always be willing to learn from those you think will make a great addition to your life. This is a mistake some people make. They let their emotions get the nest of them and choose to be envious of the person they should be learning from. I promise you that doing that wouldn't take you further than you already are.

On the other hand, you must also be willing to share information with people. Always be open to advising people who come to you for advice. You never know where an opportunity will arise from these little chit-chats.

So engage! Interact!

Figure out your Weaknesses

Career development requires you to be willing to improve every day. Find out what you stink at and your weak point, and correct yourself when you receive negative feedback. Except you don't have the passion for whatever career path, you're on, which makes you not fit for it.

Constantly fix up yourself where you have observed that there is a loophole, and with time, you'll become what you could have never imagined.

Be Yourself, Always

You cannot be another person and succeed in your career development. The moment you start pretending to be what you're not, you start losing the authenticity which makes you who you indeed are. You begin to lose your brand to someone else and trust me, that'll be the beginning of the end for you.
Life is a movie; it always plays you.

POSITIVE CAREER AFFIRMATIONS

1. My career is mine alone, and I'll create it.
2. I'm always open to new opportunities
3. I work excellently well; others can testify.
4. People enjoy working with me
5. I don't know it all; I will ask for help when needed.
6. When people come to me for help, I will help them
7. Learning never ends; I will continue to learn.
8. Bring on any challenge! I'm all for it.

9. I will work hard to get what I want.
10. I set goals, and I achieve them
11. A lot of people can't do without me.
12. I will encounter problems, and I will turn them into experiences
13. I make mistakes that I'll certainly learn from.
14. There's so much to be done that I will start working on them
15. Nothing is going to hold me back!
16. I'm going to be nothing but myself
17. I'm going to live my dreams!
18. People may think I'm crazy; I don't mind anyway; I am.
19. I'm grateful to be where I have reached so far
20. I am looking forward to and working towards a better future.
21. I am creative and competent
22. I do not take my work ethic for granted
23. I am confident in my skills and abilities
24. I have to offer something that the rest of the world can't.
25. I am fully responsible for my career success and will take the credit for it
26. I am capable of achieving the impossible
27. I find so much joy in pursuing my career, and it shows all over
28. I have the skills and talents to compete in whatever field I find myself
29. I get closer to where I want to be every day
30. I will always feel the support around me rather than the negativity.
31. I will build my career excellently.
32. I will reach the apex of my career.
33. I am the best at what I do.
34. I achieve my career goals with ease and elegance.
35. I am not deterred by the challenges I face in my career.
36. I pursue and achieve excellence with ease.

KEY POINTS

1. It would help if you did not allow yourself to settle for whatever comes at you.
2. Accept challenges
3. Your career is yours, don't give it to someone else
4. Learning is crucial to career development
5. Always have an eye on your goals.

CHAPTER EIGHT

THE WOMAN LEADER

"If your actions create a legacy that inspires others to dream more, learn more, do more, and become more, then, you are an excellent leader."
—Dolly Parton

She can become anything she has made up her mind to be. She is not held within the confines of where society wants her to be. She can be a lawyer, a surgeon, a pilot, or an engineer, and she can also be a leader.

Gone are the days when we couldn't see this happen, or even when we did, it was too strange to believe. Big ups to the individuals who have worked tirelessly to pave the way for women to rise to the task, to take on anything that arose before them, and own up to their realities rather than shying away from the world because of what it says.

It's a beautiful sight to behold, and the many who feel triggered by seeing women spread their wings need to be checked for sure. Because as long as you have worked so hard to achieve a specific goal, I see absolutely no reason why it should be denied of you because you're a woman. That's just all shades of unfair. And life is already unfair; let's not make it hard for people who try.

People who have proven themselves have to be recognized! Male or female! So it's refreshing to see women doing excellently well in their various endeavors, and that's including leadership.
So shall we?

WHO IS A LEADER?

Defining a leader from the surface perspective, I would say a leader is a person who directs a particular set of people, which could be in the form of an organization, a business enterprise, a religious group, and so on.

But the word "direct" is where the true definition of a leader lies, and it is more than just a single definition. In short, being a leader encompasses so many qualities and attributes. Most of which one must fulfill to be regarded as a true leader.

As we progress, I will be talking about some of these characteristics and qualities, but before then, I'd give a more precise definition than the one I shared previously.

A leader is a person who has a social influence on others and maximizes their efforts towards actualizing a particular goal. I think that's a more comprehensive definition, or don't you think so?

Well, if you still need clarity, there's more to come as we will be discussing a leader's characteristics right away.

QUALITIES OF A LEADER

A Sense of Purpose

If a person who is acclaimed to be a leader has no sense of purpose, then one might want to question the credibility of his leadership. Because who is a leader without a goal? If a leader lacks purpose, where are they leading the followers too? I wouldn't even know. As human beings, if we're not constantly seeing enough reasons why we're undertaking a specific task, there's a tendency that we will derail soon enough.

That is why a leader needs to have a sense of purpose, to incorporate it into his followers' minds constantly.

It helps make the day-to-day process more purposeful, which in turn helps sustain team motivation and personal investment in more significant goals. A leader without a sense of purpose cannot achieve this and shouldn't even be leading in the first place unless he makes improvements.

Empathy

I have observed that most people see leaders as unapproachable and inaccessible. It immensely saddens me because it is what we see today which has been implanted in the minds of the general public.

A leader is far from that. A leader should not just be accessible; he must be able to empathize with their team members. It spurs them up to go out of their way to ensure they carry out their responsibilities diligently and do so without grudges.

By listening to their subordinates and being open about their appreciation for their teams, a sense of value is imparted to the group by the leaders. When people feel valued, it makes them happy, and they tend to do more of what they have appreciated. When leaders prioritize empathy and acknowledge their team members' efforts, they can empower team members to see the vision for themselves and work hard toward its achievement.

Leaders, putting themselves in the position of their team members with a sense of understanding, also help to address critical concerns of the subordinates and provide solutions.

Vision

There's always a bigger picture to be seen behind every goal. This vision makes it almost impossible for a short-sighted person to be a leader.

Leaders should be able to see the bigger picture and forge unity with their team members behind their vision. By incorporating team strengths and core values, a leader inspires their team with the results at the tail end that resonate with individual values and prompt action.

The vision has to be, however, aligned with the organization's core values, or else the work channeled towards the organization's progress may fall shy. One doesn't just have to stay afloat; there should be progress. Without progress, little or nothing is achieved at the end of the day, and with all the energy channeled in the wrong direction, progress may not be achieved.

Creativity

As a leader, you have to be creative and innovative in tackling whatever problems may arise in the course of your leadership. You may have devised a particular way of solving problems but sticking to the status quo for a long time is risky. Times are changing, and the world is evolving rapidly. There is always a need to revolve with it, even taking risks.

You might want to play it safe by sticking to the good old days when there were many new things to be done. You don't realize that the competition is fierce, and you must be as bright as possible to beat your peers.

That won't be healthy for you and your subordinates, who may try their best but get frustrated because they see little or no results.

Motivation

Leaders ought to be good motivators and create goals that align with the organization's values to inspire team members to work toward the company's vision. Coupled with reaching out consistently, leaders empower their team members to work passionately beyond their responsibilities to achieve a common objective.

I must say this. Motivation is not all about inspiring words; you can motivate your subordinates by listening to whatever question they have and whatever idea they have to bring to the table. It gives your followers a sense of belonging and incorporates a sense of leadership in them.

Making Room for Improvement

As a leader, you should never stop trying to find a better version of yourself daily. Aiming for growth, leaders continuously look for opportunities to make improvements for themselves and their teams. This leaning towards personal gain means leaders should always seek feedback and value ideas that favor effectiveness and progress instead of trying to defend their egos.

When leaders create an enabling environment for feedback that isn't just helpful but highly valued, it is a source of inspiration for team members to speak their thoughts and bring the best ideas to the table. This can bring about higher innovation, leading to long-term success.

Communication

I'd speak on this lastly.

A leader who doesn't communicate with us is no leader at all. Because they wouldn't be able to do much of what we've previously spoken about.
Good leaders must be able to communicate with their followers in a way that feels genuine. This does not mean it's a must to be an extrovert or a leader. Many great leaders have identified themselves as introverts! Instead, it means exhibiting empathy, as we discussed before, engaging in active listening, and building meaningful working

relationships with those around you, whether they are a peer or a direct report.

Out of so many, these are the few qualities one must possess to be considered a leader. It's so much more than giving orders and overseeing the activities of an organization.

There are several misconceptions about leadership I would like to bring to your knowledge—just a few before we move on.

I'd like to name this topic;

LEADERSHIP MISCONCEPTIONS

We will discuss under this topic what leadership is not to enable you to make your distinctions.

Let's move on.

First of all, leadership had nothing to do with age. Many people make this mistake, and it's high time it stopped.

I need you to rule out such expectations from your minds! You might be shocked at the reality, ladies! Not to sound too harsh, but fools grow old too. Attaining a certain age doesn't make you a leader above those who haven't. You may have a certain level of experience, but that doesn't automatically bestow the mantle of leadership on you. If you still think like that, you need to grow up! Wake up to reality! The administration has not and will never be based on age.

Leadership has nothing to do with your position in an organization. It doesn't matter what hierarchy you are in in your organization; if you're not a leader, that position will not grant you leadership. Let's get that into our heads now. Too many people talk about an organization's leadership and reference the senior-most executives in the organization. The plain truth is, they are nothing more than that, senior executives and not leaders. When you reach a certain level in your company, leadership is not automatically bestowed on you. Maybe you can find your feet as a leader there, but there are no guarantees.

Thirdly, leadership has nothing to do with titles. I know many things about leadership, and one thing I'm a hundred percent sure of is that leadership is not about what name you're called.

You can be a leader in your place of worship, your neighborhood, and your family without a title.

And finally, leadership has nothing to do with personal attributes or characteristics. I don't want this to sound strange to you. Many people have often associated personality traits with leadership, but I'm here to tell you that it doesn't play so much a role.

Think of a leader, and so many minds trace to an authoritative figure who loves giving orders and ensures they're carried out or an extroverted personality like I earlier mentioned.

No! That's not what leadership entails.

Extroverted charismatic traits are not needed to practice leadership. And those with charisma don't automatically become leaders.

WOMEN IN LEADERSHIP

Now that we've spoken at length about what leadership is about from the general perspective, how about we be a little more exact?

Women in Leadership roles. What does this prospect bring to the table? One might ask.

I want to start by stating that there are always two sides to everything—the advantageous and the disadvantageous.

But you ladies should know me by now; I'm here to blow your horns! For all I care, you're the best and nothing but the best, so all I've got to say about you is the excellent part: even in your imperfections, you're perfect!

So back to the question of the moment.

What does the prospect of women in leadership bring to the table? In other words, why should women lead? What leadership qualities do they naturally possess that can make them a good pick for the team? It's going to be a long stretch; I hope you stick with me through the ride.

Value for Balance

What I mean by balance here is the one between work and life. Or I'd say, Work-Life balance for short. I think women tend to understand better that there is a life outside the organization they are in control of, so it wouldn't be much of a problem when they're approached by, let's say, a subordinate, making a personal request other than work-life. The understanding women often possess for work-life balance places them on a different level in leadership, making it more enjoyable to be led by them.

They are More Empathetic

One of the qualities of leadership we discussed earlier is empathy, and it is common knowledge that when it comes to that, a large percentage of women will be above their male counterparts.

Some people mistake the empathetic nature of women for weakness. They believe that to be a leader, one must be aggressive or assertive. But that's far from the truth, ladies. Don't you ever let anyone tell you that you're wealthy because you choose not to be a dragon?

I'll forever refuse to agree that you cannot be both strong and compassionate. Never!

Great Multitaskers

Women are naturally good at multitasking, and that isn't even a debate. From the onset, everyone should know that. Multitasking is a trait that women possess, and even if just multitasking will never be enough, it counts.

The ability to give decisive and quick responses to simultaneous and different tasks or problems at a time is vital to being a successful leader.

Better Communicators

A more significant percentage of women communicate better. I honestly do not want to make all these sound like a debate, but I can't seem to help it.

Be it communication with employers, co-workers, or partners, women know how to use this tool excellently well. As we've previously discussed, a communication stream allows for clarity in carrying out duties and responsibilities. Female leaders can already communicate regularly, clearly, and openly. And believe it or not, this is a big plus to whatever organization or team they manage.

Flexibility

This quality is often overlooked when it comes to leadership, and it marvels me. Rigidity makes it hard for people to evolve. You'll be left behind because you're too busy still trying out your old-fashioned practices and wondering why things aren't going as smoothly as they used to be.

Anyways, women are more open to new ideas from people and would likely waste no time in implementing those ideas. Especially when they notice that the system they had formerly adopted is no longer working as it used to.

Inclusiveness

I believe that the male and the female gender naturally have different ways of approaching certain things. Wouldn't you agree with me? I guess you would.
With our concern being leadership, I'd say that women tend to be more inclusive, they reach out more, and they care a little more.

A necessary attribute to possess as a leader is the ability to carry everyone along. And I think that women have the upper hand on this one.

Emotional Intelligence

Emotional intelligence is the ability to recognize the emotions in yourself and that in others and relate. It's like putting your legs in someone else's shoes to try to understand certain things you would not ordinarily understand. And it is something that has recently gained cognizance as a vital leadership attitude.

I also firmly believe that this comes more naturally to women than men. (Trust me, ladies, I'm trying my best not to make this look like a debate)

But to be honest, I have experienced this several times, so yeah, I'd agree with that. To truly create a great place to work and to get the best out of subordinates, exhibiting emotional intelligence as a leader is crucial and should not be overlooked.

Ability to Handle Crises

Many women, especially mothers, are naturally trained caretakers who know how to deal with crises at home with so much compassion and patience. These qualities are very relevant when a woman leader deals with problems relating to her subordinates.

Defying the Odds

Lastly, women make great leaders because of the circumstances surrounding their ambitions. It's not a piece of new information that the odds are always stacked up against women being in leadership positions. So when you see a woman at the top, you should know that it took more than the average for her to get there. You know when you're the underdog, it's going to take a little more than the norm to get to the top.

The challenges women face and overcome in their journey to leadership make them extraordinarily strong and capable.

They had to fight so hard to get there!

It is no doubt that from the onset, women's leadership has been revolutionary, and they have made a huge impact wherever they find themselves at the top. Well, this is to tell you that you can defy the odds too and become a great black women leader who is proud of her heritage and will put in the necessary work to achieve the best results.

You are extraordinary women who encompass these values and even more and will make great leaders wherever.

I want to let you know that you're killing it wherever you go; you are limitless, full of strength and vigor, capable of being what you want and not what people have said you are.

Never afraid and never relenting, you are the epitome of the woman leader!

POSITIVE AFFIRMATIONS FOR LEADERSHIP

1. I am a natural leader
2. I am proud of my team, and they're also proud of me.
3. I am willing to explore new ideas.
4. I communicate skillfully.
5. People are aware of where they stand with me.
6. People achieve unbelievable heights under my leadership
7. I welcome the opinions of others
8. Challenges energize me.
9. I love to see my team succeed.
10. I have faith in my leadership skills
11. I never stop improving my leadership skills
12. My leadership is flexible
13. I'm an inspiration to my followers
14. I always see the bigger picture
15. I run with a sense of purpose
16. I will always bring out the best in my team
17. I respect my colleagues, and they respect me too
18. Challenges don't and will never deter me
19. I am a leader with knowledge and understanding
20. I feel great when I see my team excel
21. I become a better leader with every passing day.
22. I can handle failure and will forgive myself for the mistakes
23. I judge the situation well and make excellent decisions
24. I am willing to step out of my comfort zone
25. I am a model for my followers to emulate
26. I don't need to prove anything to anyone but myself
27. I am not afraid of taking calculated risks
28. I am confident that teams need leaders like me to move forward
29. It will never happen that I give up on my team

30. I am not going to disappoint all those who believe in my abilities
31. I will not be a partial leader.
32. I embrace quality leadership with the whole of my being.
33. I am not a despotic leader; I lead with wisdom and fairness.
34. My subjects listen to me.
35. I am surrounded by issues that make leadership easy.
36. I was born to be a great leader.
37. My leadership is a blessed one.

KEY POINTS

1. Being a leader is not dependent on age or position
2. Women in leadership are revolutionary
3. Leadership is not only about giving orders
4. A leader should be empathetic
5. One has to strive to be a better leader every day.

CHAPTER NINE

THE BLACK WOMAN AND BEAUTY

"There is no definition of beauty, but when you can see someone's spirit coming through, something unexplainable, that's beautiful to me."
-Liv Tyler

The fact that after having the worst day of one's life, one will still find himself sleeping for hours like the worst didn't just happen is beautiful. What is beauty? Who is beautiful? Who is the beholder?

Whenever the word 'Beauty' is mentioned in any article or gathering, any place at all, the first thing I think about is that it's relative. Oh, yes, beauty is undoubtedly close to physicality. It means that I could find a diastema attractive and a dimple unattractive.

When it comes to the physical attributes of a person, then beauty varies from person to person. But it would be utterly vain if beauty was attributed only to the aesthetics of a person and not what was in their heart, how they behaved and treated others.

This is why whenever I'm talking or writing about the black woman and beauty, I always go both ways, the physical and inner beauty.

Beauty is like art (it is art, in fact); it owes no explanation; experience got nothing on it; knowledge is even let down; consciousness is shifted to the subconscious- one can only be attracted, not by one of the senses(sight) but, all.

The black woman is a woman, a shade of women. Do you know that black is all the colors put together in one? Black possesses all the charm, splendor, spark, and thrill, but it is always considered dark at one glance.

BEAUTY

General Overview of Beauty

We've established that physical beauty is relative. For a general understanding of beauty, you, my dear black woman, should note that beauty has subjective and objective aspects. That is, it can be perceived as subjectively based on the feelings of people, the opinions they hold, or even their tastes, and objective-based on a property of things. The subjective aspect of beauty is why people say, *"Beauty is in the eye of the beholder."* To date, we do not have an account of who the beholder is, so we can trace that generation to be the judge and pass a verdict on who is beautiful. But that is true, but I'll tell you this: the beholder has always been with you from day one, always standing close to you, walking with and begging for your attention all this while. You should know now that the beholder is the person you see when you look at your reflection. Do you appreciate your body, struggles, dreams, and status? Do you look back and look at yourself now and admire just how far you've come?

Black woman! To become beautiful, you must be attracted to yourself first. When you are, the world will see how total you are. To be black means to have survived; it was never easy for you, the world was challenging, and you had to be harsh or more demanding, which is the foundation of your beauty. That means you are strong; look at your skin and smile sometimes *"Hey, rhino, nothing can mar or impel you."*

Check out gold- it takes all that heat to become the sparkly thing we all know, and you know you can't just pick it up quickly; you'll have to spend big. Think that! You're rare, remarkable; you're beautiful without even trying.

BEAUTY; THE INSECURITY

Hey girl, you've been staring at that magazine for quite a while now, and I see that you do that almost every time I walk by your house in the morning and evening. What exactly are you looking at that you cannot just take your eyes off the pieces of paper? Let me have a look. Kim Kardashian, Beyonce, and Rihanna look so beautiful in these magazines. But I just stared at those pictures for a minute, and I already don't see the need to look over and over any longer.

Are you sure you only find them beautiful? Or is there something else to it?

Hello, young lady. Anytime I drop by to visit a friend, you're always tuned to Entertainment News on the TV. Most of the time, I believe they repeat shows, and I must have seen you more than twice, watching the same show. Don't you get bored or something? I'm a little bit concerned, you know. What's going on?

I can tell that these two ladies have passed the stage of admiration as they absorb the contents of the magazine and the screen, respectively.

The look in their eyes. It is no more extended admiration. The eyes have changed, and the excitement has disappeared from their faces like the evening sun setting into the clouds.

They're no longer admiring the stars; they're now disgusted by themselves, and their look is revealed to me.

"She looks so perfect! Look at her eyes, her skin, smooth as the moon! Her perfectly rounded face gave me goosebumps the first time I saw them on TV, but now, I feel so horrible that I could never achieve such a feat." One of them said, *"Can you see how skinny I look? Just take a look at the woman in the magazine! Those curves are a representation of heaven on earth! I want to be like she is! Why have I even created this way? I'm fed up!"*

Beauty insecurity can make a mental mess of most women these days, and I wish I had a magic wand that could bring everything to an end with just one swing.

Because it's not worth it! Most of the time, what they see in magazines and TV shows isn't even real. These people have significantly benefited from make-up artists and surgeons to make them look good, and you're letting them cause unnecessary pain and fuel your insecurities.

That's just too bad, and to make it worse, society has also set standards for beauty, which are having horrible effects on women every day, leading to more horrible consequences, a few of which will be discussed below.

Low Self-Esteem

Every woman who takes these beauty standards to heart and falls short in one way or the other tends to suffer from low self-esteem.

For instance, when society has declared a specific style old-fashioned, many people who have no choice but to stick to those trends will likely suffer low self-esteem any time they walk down the road. They don't want to be scapegoats. They don't want to get home at the end of the day, open up Twitter and see that there are already numerous pictures of them taken unaware, and then they have to be the laughing stock of the day.
And nobody even seems to care! Well, I do. I'm one of those who believe that you are beautiful just the way you are. If you feel like trying other ways of improving your physical looks by working out, or something of that sort, it'll only be a matter of choice for such a person and not necessarily because they have low self-esteem.

Overthinking

So many people can stay up late at night, thinking about how their lives have turned out with the kind of body they have and thinking about how their lives could have been if they had the perfect body instead.

Also, people who have been abused because of their appearance are victims of overthinking. And as they think, they begin to ask themselves questions like, why don't I have the body the society wants? They begin to compare themselves with others and start amplifying their imperfections. Overthinking then leads to the following side effect.

Self-Condemnation

Every day you wake up, you're even afraid to look in the mirror because you're not good enough for your eyes to see. And if you stand in the mirror, it is to backlash yourself. And to tell yourself that you look ugly and that there's no redemption for you.
I thought we were supposed to be our number one fan, but now the standards that society has denied many people that privilege.

Self-Isolation

I think this should follow after self-condemnation. You don't want to be among your peers any more because you feel they don't like you and judge you, which could be false.

You turn down outings and cancel appointments to ensure that you're not seen among your perfect-looking peers because you feel that their appearances will always find a way to accentuate your imperfections. As a result, you could miss out on so many opportunities that may arrive just because you didn't want to come outside because you hate how you look.

What a flimsy excuse that is!

Desperation

Probably fed up with what you're passing through, you decide that you need to change the narrative soon and that you need to do every single thing possible for you to get what you want.

You can even go as far as implanting artificial body parts to make sure you look good and accepted, knowing fully well that these things have side effects and have caused the death of some people in the past; you don't seem to care, you want to look good, and that'll make you happy.

According to society's standards, you look too thin, take weight gain pills, eat unhealthily, excessively, which may turn into an eating disorder, so many things! To make sure you're in the shape society wants you to be. I wish you don't care, but as it stands, I do not have a say.

In addition, most of these activities you carry out to change the structure of your body have massive side effects on the body, and when the side effects start coming in, you are plagued with trying to make things look better, all to no avail. And your life may never be the same.

That's to show how society's standards can endanger the lives of humans if not properly grounded.
So then, how can we be free from whatever bondage society has made for us?

What steps to take to make you feel good about yourself again?

Let's have some;

Exercise Daily

Taking part in exercise routines is a perfect way to get back in good shape and live a healthier lifestyle. This will not only make you look better physically, but it also ensures that your mental health improves. There are so many benefits of breaking a sweat that you'd be silly not to include exercise in your day-to-day activities. The only way to overcome your beauty insecurities is to face the challenges head-on and not be afraid of the little hard work, as that's a small price to pay for salvation.

If you don't feel too good about how your body is right now, you have to take this chance to step up and make the necessary improvements to the areas that disturb you the most.

Skin and Haircare, Manicure, and Pedicure

Especially as a woman, your beauty routine has to include paying attention to your skin, hair, and nails if you want to look and feel your best. These basic things play a massive role in defining your beauty. For example, washing your face regularly and searching for products that help you take care of any blemishes or dry skin will help you feel more confident in your skin. Your hair, too, is golden. You must learn to care for it or even develop a particular routine to ensure it is always kept in check. Care for your hair by going to the salon regularly and getting the ends trimmed to keep them looking ever fresh and pleasant. In addition, you also have to do well too, get your nails done, or, if you can, do them yourself at home and apply fun and fresh color that makes a statement and gives you the confidence boost you need. You'll feel like a new person if you consistently give yourself the attention you deserve in these three beauty areas.

Go Shopping

One reason a person could feel insecure about how they look is due to their wardrobe. By that, I mean what's in it. If what they own is old-fashioned and outdated and they're finding it hard to find anything to wear, then there's a tendency that they could feel frustrated and unattractive.

First, you need to start by cleaning your closet and removing or donating what you no longer need or wear. Afterward, head online or to the stores to select a few new garments and outfits that will make you feel great and comfortable and complement your figure nicely.

As a young lady, I always went through this routine every few months to keep up with the changing seasons and styles. This is very important.

Keep Records

One significant but easy way to get in better tune with yourself and your insecurities is bordered on is to pen it down in a journal so you can tackle them one after the other. It looks basic but tries it, makes a list, and see with your two eyes what's being the source of disturbance to you or your mind so you can take action. Always record what you don't like and then devise a list of possible solutions to get past and work through your insecurities. Trust me; you don't want to find yourself constantly complaining about what bothers you and then going ahead and doing nothing about it. That's just a waste of paper and pen ink. Always make sure to use your journal as a reality check and write down all you love about yourself and why you're beautiful.

Share with Others

Now, this doesn't mean calling others for their pity, as there's absolutely nothing wrong with opening up to others, especially your friends, about your beauty insecurities and seeking some advice from the outside. You may never know; someone may have suggestions that will significantly help you or allow you to observe your imperfections from a whole new point of view. Search for a trusted friend, family member, or therapist in whom you can confide and who will be willing to listen and give some feedback and advice to you if you're receptive to it. You may find that many others struggle with some of the same insecurities and that you're not alone on this journey.

To conclude, let us not forget that no one's perfect, so you don't have to be either. You will always dislike that part of your body as much as others. However, you have to be open to overcome these insecurities and appreciate what you have going for you that you love. It is all about building your confidence and getting comfortable in your skin. Don't give up until you reach a point where you're able to walk around with your head held high, queen!

Black Beauty

In the past, society did a lot to trample upon black women and women in general, setting high standards to what it meant to be beautiful, and being black was not among them.

If you were chubby, had a physical defect, with kinky hair, or the like, you weren't fit to be called beautiful. Over the years, black women have begun to stand on their feet and say, "guess what, we are the ones with our bodies, and we get to decide if it's beautiful or not, not anyone, not even society!"

Oh yes, that's the spirit I see in every black woman I come across, the radiance, the self-confidence reeking like perfume from around them; it gladdens my heart so much that I cannot help but support this cause.

Blackness is more than just one thing; it's not a monolith where you talk about a single skin tone, hair textures, facial features, or the like. It encompasses multiple skin tones, hair textures, and beauty rituals. Black people are taking back their places in retail spaces and beauty brands. I love to see black women sharing their definitions of beauty as opposed to what the society they come from thinks about them. No one knows you better than you know yourself, so I don't expect you to believe some propaganda a group of people brews up against you when you see within yourself that it isn't true.

This section is about black beauty and owning up to it. For you to be considered a black beauty, it's not necessarily about having glowing caramel, olive skin, or even a copious amount of melanin, dear black woman. Black beauty is about confidence in your dark skin, even its flaws. It's walking up shoulder high and saying to those who try to shame you that despite the massive scar on your face, despite the brown skin that seems to set you aside from the whites and blacks, you don't care about any of it, and you're beautiful just as you are.

One of my close friends from Zimbabwe has this attitude I love so much. Her skin is so dark, and she cares so much for it, applies oil and lotions, goes to the spa often, you know, all of that skincare just because she is so in love with her skin tone. Now, I'm not saying you must apply all the lotions in the world before you're sure you love your skin, far from it. To love your skin is to be proud, show it to the world, and forget about your insecurities. Everyone has theirs; take care of your body and skin, and speak positively about your skin. That's all that is required. It's that simple.

I've been reasonable to be with many black women and seized the opportunity to ask what black beauty means to them. Some say it's confident in your roots, being unapologetic despite what your white counterparts may say about you. It has to keep your head up in a society where you have to work thrice as hard to prove yourself because you're black. You know, one thing that makes people, especially the whites, want to bully black women is because they're afraid of who you are, and let them be!

If they choose to hate you because you're black, you must give them no room for breathing space; oh yes, flaunt your beauty and let them know you're not ashamed of your skin. Wear your Afro proudly, fix those extensions, dress in your traditional clothes or in your English wear, whatever you decide to do, I think what should come first is that you feel good about yourself.

I'll conclude once again that black beauty is about how you see yourself and not what people or society says about you. Rather than hate on your skin or go to the extreme to bleach it, embrace it and love it; apply Shea butter, moringa oil, or whatever is great for your skin.

I'm rooting for you, my precious black woman.

POSITIVE AFFIRMATIONS FOR BEAUTY

1. I am beautiful
2. I love myself at every time of the day
3. My imperfections make me unique
4. I accept myself in all my imperfections
5. I don't need a change to feel attractive to myself
6. I am happy and content with how I look.
7. I appreciate my beauty
8. My beauty has to be seen and appreciated
9. I am sexy and gorgeous
10. My natural look is on point
11. My smile radiates my beauty
12. I am beautiful inside out
13. I am the best of my kind
14. I have zero reasons to feel ashamed of my body
15. I love every scar, every wrinkle, every imperfection.
16. Other people's opinion of my body doesn't get to me.
17. I get complimented for my appearance all the time
18. My confidence is top-notch; it makes the difference.
19. I wake up feeling attractive every day
20. I won't give anyone the chance to make me feel bad about myself
21. The happier I am, the more beautiful I will become
22. I have a positive outlook on life and it makes me more attractive
23. I'm smashing sexy in whatever outfit I put on
24. I accept my compliments because I deserve them
25. I will achieve whatever weight loss goals I have set for myself step by step
26. My skin glows like the sun, and I'm super grateful for that
27. My smile is infectious and makes me look more beautiful

28. I am beautiful inside-out
29. I am in love with every part of my body
30. I radiate beauty from the inside.
31. Every piece of me is beautiful.

KEY POINTS

1. Beauty goes beyond physical appearance
2. Beauty never goes out of style
3. Social media is the perpetrator of harmful beauty standards
4. Insecure people set beauty standards
5. Everyone is beautiful in their way.

CHAPTER TEN

A HEALTHY MIND

"No food will ever hurt you as much as an unhealthy mind"
-Brittany Burgunder

What do you think of when you come across a title like this? Or, what does it mean for a person to have a healthy mind? Take a few seconds to think about the question I just asked and try to answer it.

Time's up! What did you find?

You might have to answer that yourself, but I'm the kind of person who always wants to believe that no one should be wrong about their own opinion. I'm more concerned with giving my two cents and hopping out as if nothing happened.

Yup! That's how I like it.

So whatever your answer was, I guess you were right about it. But give me a chance to say what I think it should be.

I'm going to try my best to try not to impose any of my opinions on anyone; it might be hard, but trust me when I say I'm going to try my best, and if in any way you feel like I'm doing that, I apologize in advance, because one can get carried away sometimes you know.

So I'm begging your pardon from the beginning, and it'll mean a lot to me if you'd remember.

Alright! Let's not waste too much time and get down to the day's business. A healthy mind, let's discuss.

THE HUMAN MIND

Before we talk about a healthy mind, it's fair to talk about the general reason and what it does. Talking about what the mind is and does isn't what should be discussed separately. I mean, talking about what the mind is saying, what it does or is responsible for. So, I won't dwell here for a long time. We do it quickly, and we move as soon as we can!

As we already know, the mind is responsible for many things going on and on in our heads. What have we? Sensation, thinking, reasoning, perception, memory, belief, motivation, desire, emotion, and confidence. Even more, I think, I can't seem to find my way around some more, but I'm sure that there's more than the mind takes care of.

I'm already finding a way to place so much importance on the subject from the beginning. I need to lay the foundation now; look at all the things I mentioned above that the mind is responsible for. They're many, and they are all critical. I have to treat all of them with care. Maybe I'm going too fast already, so I should slow down.

THE MIND IS DISSECTED

We've got three types of minds. This may sound strange, and yes, it did sound strange the first time I heard it, but I got used to it when I finally understood what it meant, and I believe you will too when I explain further.

When we talk about the mind, note that there are three significant concepts to consider deeply. These include; the conscious, subconscious, and unconscious minds.

It's something we should all be familiar with, in one way or the other. We may not see it from the same perspective, but it doesn't matter much; honestly, it's good enough that I've got a platform to share a bit of my mind with you all, which means, like, the whole world to me.

To begin, the conscious mind of any human being is the part of the mind that we are most knowledgeable about. It is the part of the mind we use in reasoning. It can be influenced more quickly than other parts of the mind. And what this means is that anyone can change their minds when presented with a compelling argument outweighing theirs.

Please don't mistake the above for vulnerability, though; it doesn't make you less of a human. It makes you more human to be easily convinced sometimes. What if you're wrong about something? Do you see? Your mind isn't always right about a particular thing and may require some convincing.

So when I say the conscious mind is easy to manipulate, don't mistake the assertion for weakness.

The conscious mind is that part of the mind you use in everyday activities. When people bring up "the mind" in conversations, most times, what they are referring to is the conscious part of it.

Next, I'll be discussing the unconscious mind. The subconscious mind is a very active part of the mind, but it is not one that you'd notice very clearly if you're not meticulous. It is the part of the mind that sees everything your conscious mind ignores, from random pieces of information to things that happened in your childhood. It picks up different selections of information and stores distant memories. Then, it brings them to your remembrance on days you do not expect.

Lastly, I'll talk about the subconscious. (Reason why I saved it for the last, I guess you didn't have to wait much longer to understand.) The subconscious mind is the most complicated and, for this discussion, the most important. It is where mental programs are formulated and carried out. If you need to change the way you think so severely, the subconscious mind is where you'll need to focus more.

There's more to be spoken about here, it's exciting, and it's something I'd love to share with you all, but I'm going to try my best not to dwell so much on it; you might get bored. So after a simple illustration, I'll be done with this.

Let's throw life back to the days we were kids for a bit.
As an adult reading this, this may sound a bit absurd, but maybe later, take a little time to analyze the illustration, and you'll see what I'm saying.

So, as I was saying, as kids or babies, we tend to find a line of relationship between particular things subconsciously. The resulting relationships drawn are solely based on experiences, and experiences differ, so what I'm trying to say in essence is that, for the same thing, backgrounds may be different, and this makes whatever relationship drawn from them differ as well.

Let's use an example, two kids who grew up in different neighborhoods. One of them lives near a pet house where dogs are all nice and squishy, and the other, an environment chokehold by crimes hence, the need for security dogs all over the place. We all know these dogs have no business with being all cute and squishy like the former. These dogs are trained to attack at the slightest knowledge of unusual activity by unusual people.

So this is how it probably starts.

The kid in the friendlier environment first hears dogs barking, and the first reaction is shocking. After that, he tries to find out where the sound had come from and discovers that it had come from a pet dog in his home. At that moment, to the kid, the only thing that can make such a sound is the harmless, strange-looking, furry, four-legged creature always running around the house, and that's what he thinks till he hears the same sound, while the dog in his place is asleep. Oh wow! How's this possible? He'd probably think to himself, but the time will come when he accepts that his furry friend isn't the only dog around. By then, he would have wholly associated the sound with the face he saw.

And then one more thing, the most important, is how his mind reacts when he hears the barking.

Since dogs don't harm people in the neighborhood, the barking he hears is not a call for alarm and could be for anything else, probably announcing its arrival or just anything else but a call for alarm.

On the other hand, I wouldn't have to explain so much. It's all the same logic but just a different environment with a different breed of dogs. And instead of seeing a cute little creature wagging its tail when the kid hears barking, it's a different scenario here in the hood.

The kid would most likely see a ferocious-looking creature with bloodshot eyes running after a person or, in a worse situation, the creature pouncing on its victim and doing whatever harm it could before it's held back. That's not sweet to see for a kid. And that's where it all starts, especially when this happens almost daily. That kid then grows to ignore the sweet side of "man's best friend" even if he is told in school by his teacher that dogs can be harmless; I don't think words of the mouth can erase the notion he has from what he has seen. It's even worse when a dog himself attacked him.

So you see, that's how the mind works in the subtlest of ways. They're both kids, but the difference in the environment has changed their notion of how they'd see the same thing.

That's why the black woman needs to be very conscious of the environment she raises her kids. I'm talking to you ladies. Even if you didn't have it quite right while growing up, you must make sure you don't make the same mistake your parents made. Black ladies are great mothers! Don't forget that!

And that's that for the subconscious mind. I hope you can see how important it is, relate the illustration with other aspects of life that can affect the mind, and take the right action where you should.

After a fair dissection of the different types of the mind, how they work, and their importance, it's time to move on to something new.

TAKING CONTROL

I have been going through a breakup, betrayal, loss of a loved one, job loss, racism, sexist situations, domestic abuse, man! There are a lot of these issues that can make a mess out of your mind. I'm supposed to talk about these things, but why ponder so much on the problem when there's a solution to be given? I'm making a bit of sense, am I not?

Anyway, while we admit that everyone goes through a lot of stuff that could make their minds a mess, we also have to acknowledge that there are solutions, and you need to do something about them.

Tell me, does it sound weird that you have to control your mind? I'm asking because it may only make sense that our minds hold us instead. These are just two contrasting opinions that may be both valid anyway.

Want to know my take on this? I would be more than delighted to let you all know. That's all I've been doing all this while, so why not?

Well, to me, it goes both ways. Your mind takes control of you, but there's a catch. You've got to take control first. In other words, whatever your mind controls you to do, is a product of whatever has been done to it (life comes at you fast, you know?) I think that makes sense. Or, maybe not yet, but as we go further, I think I should be able to make you understand. And I believe you all trust me to do all that.

So the main question here is how can one control the mind? There are many ways to do that, and we're going to explore quite a number.

Here we go!

Know What You Face

In other words, you've got to identify what thoughts you need to eliminate due to whatever life has brought your way. Maybe your ex broke up with you because he wrongly thought he had found someone more beautiful. (No one's more beautiful than you are, my black queen.)

I know it's hard not to feel that sting of low self-esteem all over the place. Now that's where you should start!

You must know what thoughts you're battling and be sure you know. At first, gaining total control of your mind could be difficult due to damage done. Or, you could be an over thinker with a sense all over the place. But despite all of these, I need you to know that gaining control of your mind is not impossible, and you shouldn't see it as such.

But you have to take the proper steps and put first things first. Taking time to learn and understand specific patterns effectively will help you make the most of other tips in this book.

Acceptance

You've been friends with your best girl since childhood, and you think you can shy away from the pain of her betrayal in a day? Come on! That's impossible!

Though it's human nature to avoid thoughts that cause distress, there are certain things we can't just avoid, and that's life. (It feels like I've said this for the 1000th time now).

I've never seen anyone overcome mental distress by avoiding the thought. So why don't you try the opposite? Ask yourself.

"Damn! I've been playing again, haven't I?" It helps, you don't know. It does!

When you dwell on those mistakes you've made and how it's making you feel, before you know it, solutions start pouring in. It also helps you keep your mind in check because you don't want to make the same mistake again, except you enjoy pain. So ladies, dwell on that pain for a while. It helps.

Switch POVs

This has to do with self-talk.

Talking to yourself during rough times does a great deal in helping to contain the negative vibes your mind tries to spread. But there's something more.
Most of us use the first-person perspective during self-talk, which isn't a bad idea at all. But you're also open to other options, you know.

How about trying the third-person perspective? Instead of saying;

"I failed again, and I feel so miserable. I've been through worse, so I can come out of this too." Why not try;

"Hey, baby girl, I know you've done it again, and I know you're feeling all shades of miserable now, but you've done so much to get over worse situations. So this shouldn't be too much of a big deal for you. Level up, girl!"

That changes the mood. I won't lie. It's like you're distancing yourself from a part of you that only feels the distress, with your bright side sitting across the table. Switching your perspective helps trick your mind into seeing yourself as another individual, giving you the distance from your hardships.

Positivity Always!

As regards mental health, this solution will always find a way to surface every issue. Never underrate the importance of staying positive, ladies!

Positive thinking will not automatically redirect whatever dart life throws at you, but it does change how you feel about it. Now I've got to remind you that thinking doesn't mean pretending everything's going well, ignoring problems, or refusing to consider helpful solutions. Not!

Instead, it is restricting your thoughts' negativity and looking out for the brightness in the most grey skies. No matter how grey it is, there is some brightness somewhere. You have to find it by looking carefully, try zeal and hope.

Therapy

Learning to control your mind is not as easy as it may seem. It's beautiful if you feel you cannot do it on your own. Do not hesitate to seek the services of a therapist whenever life overwhelms you. It is not a thing of shame; speaking up and asking for help is a thing of strength and never weakness. Take care of your mental and emotional well-being. It is essential. A therapist will do a great deal in helping you identify underlying issues and explore potential solutions.

Therapy allows you to feel all your feelings, identify them, and heal them gradually. Remember that healing is a gradual process and doesn't happen in one day. Give yourself grace, my black queen.

In conclusion, it is not impossible to gain control of your mind. You don't need psychic powers to control your mind. But it's not an easy thing either. It takes time, but you'll be okay in the end. Again, remember to give yourself grace.

POSITIVE AFFIRMATIONS FOR A HEALTHY MIND

1. I'm mentally stable
2. My mind is healthy
3. I've been through a lot, but I'm standing here still
4. I love myself more every day
5. I'm not going to run away from my problems
6. Instead of negative thoughts, I will think positively
7. Self-care is my priority
8. The challenges of today are the stepping stones for tomorrow

9. I accept that because I can't always influence things beyond my control.
10. Tough times never last; I'll see the end of it.
11. I find peace with who I am now.
12. My mistakes do not define me
13. I will not allow negative vibes to creep all over me
14. I don't know the future, but I'll be forever hopeful.
15. I'm focusing entirely on improving my mental health
16. I am loved
17. I am in control of my mind
18. I will provide the best environment for the mental well-being of my children
19. I'm happy with whatever I am right now; it can only get better.
20. I can do this.
21. My life is filled with positive people and things
22. I am creating better mental health for myself by the day
23. I accept all the positive and negative aspects of my life in good fate
24. I am always at peace with myself
25. As long as I'm alive, my journey never ends. I will keep improving
26. I choose to be happy regardless
27. I am letting go of all my insecurities
28. I will always choose actions that improve my mental health and make me happy
29. My mind cleanses itself from bad energy and negativity
30. My mind holds memories of love and happiness.
31. I see my scars as trophies.
32. Nothing will make me come undone.
33. I have a brilliant mind.

KEY POINTS

1. Environment plays a vital role in shaping the mind
2. There are three types of reasons, the conscious, unconscious, and subconscious
3. Controlling the mind is not an easy thing to do.
4. Always be aware of your mental challenges
5. The functioning of the reason is primarily a result of experience.

CHAPTER ELEVEN

BLACK WOMEN ENTREPRENEURS

"When you're an entrepreneur you have to go in feeling like you're going to be successful."
-Lillian Vernon

Not quite a while since we spoke about black women managing their finances. Now we're here again because money is in the life of everyone and shouldn't be treated lightly.

Although entrepreneurship isn't all about money, we can't be blind to the fact that money plays a role in it, so it should be recognized as one of the integral parts of entrepreneurship. So you've got to pay attention while we go through the in and out of entrepreneurship and how it can be a tool in the hands of the black woman to make life better for herself and those she loves.

So at this point, let's build around the subject until it's deemed full-fledged enough to raise important issues and their probable solutions.

So here goes.

WHO IS AN ENTREPRENEUR?

An entrepreneur is an individual responsible for creating one or more businesses. They can also be accountable for investing in already established enterprises to make profits. Entrepreneurship is the process by which the above is set up, and it involves taking a lot of risks, bearing a lot of losses, and enjoying the profits that proceed.

I feel like it's a bit different to do what I'm about to do, and at the same time, I think it's necessary.
How about we look at a few successful women entrepreneurs who we can look up to for knowledge and motivational purposes? It wouldn't be too bad to read this book and then have to know about some names to speak if you find yourselves when the subject comes up anywhere.

Just brief profiling of their lives, and we'd be done.

GISELLE KNOWLES-CARTER

Popularly known as Beyoncé, the "Halo" crooner is a singer-songwriter born on September 4, 1981; her career in the entertainment industry started in the 1990s as a teenager. Aside from being a successful entrepreneur, she has her name stamped as one of the most influential persons in American Pop Culture, selling millions upon millions of records all over the globe.
She has also signed multi-million-dollar endorsements, has her brand known as Parkwood Entertainment, Beyonce produces movies and music, and has her clothing line.

Over the years, she has garnered a lot of fame and accolades, which of notable mention include 28 Grammy Awards, 26 MTV Video Music Awards, 24 NAACP Image Awards, 31 Bet Awards, and 17 Soul Train Music Awards, making her one of the most awarded artists of all time!

In 2014, Billboard had her named as the highest-earning black musician of all time, while in 2020, she was included on time's list of 100 women who defined the last century.

I can't find the words to describe the magnitude of such achievements, man! Unbelievable, I must say!

Let's move on.

LYNDA RAE RESNICK

Lynda Rae Resnick is a successful billionaire entrepreneur and philanthropist born in 1943 in Baltimore, Maryland, US. Together with her husband and business partner, Stewart Resnick, they facilitate several companies worthy of mention, including POM Wonderful, Fiji Water, Wonderful Halos, Wonderful Pistachios, and The Telefloral Company through their holding company known as The Wonderful Company. The company currently boasts of annual revenues exceeding 4 billion dollars.

Interesting right? Something to note. She runs the business with her hubby! While that's very sweet if you ask me, many people these days are against women having to do anything with men to assert a certain level of equality or superiority over men. Don't get wrong, I'm not against Feminism as it may seem, but people have a specific idea about it that doesn't resonate with my reasoning. You don't have to treat men as enemies to assert a particular position that society currently clamors for.

I hope society realizes there isn't a need for a gender war. It's very unnecessary.

OPRAH WINFREY

Oprah is a household name worldwide as she is considered the most powerful woman in the entertainment industry and one of its most famous black entrepreneurs. Yeah, she's black, and she's killing it!

Oprah Winfrey, born January 29, 1954, in Mississippi, U.S, is a successful actress, talk show host, philanthropist, entrepreneur, and author. She rose to be where she is from a very humble beginning.
Best known for her talk show, The Oprah Winfrey Show, broadcast from Chicago, which was the highest-rated television program of its kind in history and ran on national TV for a 25-year period of 1986 to 2011, she was also named the wealthiest African-American of the 20th century, was at a time the only black billionaire on the planet and arguably the greatest black philanthropist in history of the United States. By the year 2007, she was sometimes ranked as the most influential woman in the globe.

I know this information is what everyone knows, but it sounds new every time. A perfect example to black women and women of all racial backgrounds, Winfrey continues to use her success to launch brands and build awareness worldwide.

MADAME C.J. WALKER

She was best known as America's first Black female self-made millionaire, as recorded by the Guinness Book of World Records. A daughter of formerly enslaved people, Walker worked in a barbershop for only $1.50 a day before she created a homemade remedy that helped her hair regrow after suffering a scalp condition.

Born December 23, 1867, Walker made her fortune by developing and marketing a line of cosmetics and hair care products for black women through the business she founded, Madam C. J. Walker Manufacturing Company. She also became known for being a philanthropist and activist. She died on December May 25, 1919.

DANA ELAINE OWENS

If you know her, you'd be aware that she's a model, actress, and musician but do you know she's also an entrepreneur? Well, if you don't, that's a take-home for you.

Nicknamed Queen Latifah, she partly owns Flavor Unit Entertainment, a production company specializing in television, movies, and artist management. She was born in Newark, New Jersey, U.S, on March 18, 1970.

If it were up to me to go on, I wouldn't even be able to exhaust the list of names I've got, and you probably all know. Many black women worldwide are making headlines with prominent figures in dollars, and that one should be inspired.

Have you thought that you can't be more? Has anyone told you can't be more? Have you told yourself you can't be more? Well, maybe you should have a rethink.

I hope you enjoyed your way around some of the few women who have made it big in the entrepreneurial world. Well, I did, too; if you ask me, it's always fun talking about issues like this and inspiring too!

Moving on, we're going to explore a few types of entrepreneurship, and I'd like to break them down into four types.
Let's look at them one after the other;

SMALL BUSINESSES

As the name connotes, these businesses are small and typically don't have any intention of becoming a chain or franchise. Firms like these include restaurants, retail stores, dry cleaners, daycares, and self-employed individuals. Most of the time, people in charge of small businesses make use of their own money to get things started and only make a profit if they are successful in their venture.

SCALABLE STARTUPS

These kinds of businesses attempt to rise quickly and become profitable full-fledged companies. These ventures are less joint than small businesses. However, these startups are more likely to gain a lot of attention when they become successful than small businesses. These are the kinds of companies you hear about, started in an attic, a garage, a dorm room, or a study room on campus, as an idea thrown around by two friends who decided to act on those ideas.

These small-scale concepts may be the talk of the century, gaining investors and enabling them to grow and scale up. Most people think of this when they hear "startup" or "entrepreneur," and they envision companies like Microsoft, Amazon, or Silicon Valley.

INTRAPRENEURSHIP

This type of entrepreneurship usually occurs like a breakout from a more significant and stable establishment. A lot of times, when entrepreneurs work for a larger organization as an employee, there's a possibility that they'd see the potential to kick off new products or services that take on a life of their own. These people we now call intrapreneurs wield an entrepreneurial mindset to use the resources their current employer has made available to them. These people tend to think outside the box and continue to proffer solutions to potential problems for current and future customers. This model allows entrepreneurs to get things up and run, and it's all thanks to the support from a larger establishment.

SOCIAL ENTREPRENEURSHIP

Humans create specific societal issues and sometimes call for creative community-based solutions.

This is where social entrepreneurs take advantage of the situation by trying to create a positive change with their actions. They do this by establishing an initiative or what we call a non-profit organization, whose primary objective is to provide help to people and not make profits; these people strive to be the change they want to see in society, and their activities are centered around topics that focus on racial justice, gender inequality, environmental conservation, or serving abandoned communities in one way or another.
I believe they're other kinds of entrepreneurship, but these are a few that we can all relate to. As you read through, which one of these kinds of entrepreneurship interested you the most? Not everyone will be an entrepreneur in the end,

but I don't see why you shouldn't venture into one if you have a passion for it.

Start wherever you can, there's so much to be explored in the world, and you can be part of it if you want to.

WHAT DOES IT TAKE TO BE AN ENTREPRENEUR?

Like I said earlier, not everyone can be an entrepreneur, and some make attempts, but it's hard to say that they unfortunately fail. Yeah, I understand that the passion is there; many people have the power, but when there's a but, it's always pretty hard to navigate the hurdles one will face.

Certain qualities are required to have as a budding entrepreneur to be able to make a name out of their passion.

Here are some qualities you should have as a woman wanting to make a name as an entrepreneur in whatever field you want to venture into.

PASSION

To me, this is the main attribute of an entrepreneur. Without passion, I don't think anything can work out fine. All other qualities exist to fuel that passion you have for a sure thing. Your work has to be your passion. Because you tend to enjoy whatever you're doing and stay highly motivated when you have the power for such. It serves as a driving force, and with that force, you're motivated to do whatever it takes to be better.

It is a passion that enables you to put in those extra hours in your office or deprive yourself of sleep which can or may make a difference. Like I said before, there are hurdles to go through at the start of every entrepreneurial venture or any venture. Even with certain privileges you may have, your passion plays the most significant role in ensuring that you can overcome these hindrances and forge ahead towards your goal.

KNOWLEDGE

Whatever prospect you wish to venture in, knowledge will always play a key role in facilitating its success.
As an entrepreneur, you must possess considerable knowledge of your field of interest. How would you be able to solve specific problems that you would encounter without knowledge? Only with the understanding that a difficulty can be tackled or a crisis resolved.

Knowing enables you to be aware of the developments and the constant changes occurring in the field in which you are based. It could be a new trend in the fashion industry that many fashion enthusiasts are making quite a fortune from or advancement in technology that makes a particular activity in your field of interest easier to navigate. As an entrepreneur, you should keep abreast of such knowledge as you will be left behind while others move forward.

Passion drives you, but knowledge guides you to leave the competition behind. New bits and pieces of information may prove as helpful as a newly devised strategy, and you will most likely be on the wrong side of the tide without being aware of it.

RISK-TAKING

You'll be an average businesswoman if you can't take risks.

Why settle for average? The black woman can always do more. I have a lot of faith in you.

The truth is, without the will to venture into the unknown, it is impossible to discover something special and unique. And without a doubt, uniqueness is what makes all the difference if you ask me.
I don't want to sound like risk-taking is an easy job; it involves a lot of things.

Using unorthodox methods is a risk. Investing in ideas nobody believes in, but you are also a risk! It takes a lot of willpower to do such things, but it might be worth it in the end! In addition, entrepreneurs must have a well-calculated approach to risks. Promising entrepreneurs will always be ready to invest their time and money. But, they always have a backup plan for every chance they take if their plan doesn't work out as expected. That's where weighing the odds comes into play.

Evaluation of the risk to be undertaken is essential. A good entrepreneur won't risk it all if he doesn't know the consequences. Never forget.

PLANNING

A school of thought may consider this quality the most important of all steps needed to make a great entrepreneur. I agree with them, but I'll still take my passion for it. However, you still have to recognize that it's difficult for anything to fall into place without planning. You know what they say, "If you fail to plan, you plan to fail." It's that simple.
Planning is simply laying out the whole game ahead of time. It is a summation of all the available resources that allows

you to devise a framework for how to reach your desired goal.

Then apart from planning, you also have to make maximum use of the resources you've used in planning. Confronting a crisis with a plan will always be better. It provides you with the guidelines with little or no damages to be incurred.

PROFESSIONALISM

It is one quality that's less talked about, to be honest. And that's sad because it is a quality all promising entrepreneurs must possess but sadly, it's always overlooked. An entrepreneur's mannerisms and attitude towards whoever they work with will go a long way in developing their organization's culture.

Alongside the attribute of professionalism is reliability and self-discipline, which plays a vital role in helping an entrepreneur reach their targets; as an entrepreneur, never forget to be organized and set an example for everyone looking up to you.

When you're reliable, it results in many people trusting your ability. For most ventures, trust in the entrepreneur keeps the people he serves locked in and whatever work he has in the organization motivated and willing to put in their best.

Trust me, ladies, professionalism is one of the essential characteristics of an entrepreneur.

I honestly wish I could go on and on because the list is inexhaustible. But I think this is also a proper place to stop, or isn't it? I hope it is for my queens; they mean a lot to me, and I'd let them know whenever I have the opportunity.

Well, I want to draw the curtain close here, there are many more exciting topics to discuss, and I honestly can't wait to share them with you. However, you know I'd never leave you without the affirmations, don't you?

I honestly wish you could feel how I feel having this little talk with you ladies. I feel blessed, and I wish I could do this forever.

That's how much you all mean to me, ladies.

AFFIRMATIONS

1. I attract success
2. I am willing to get to know about new things every day
3. I'm ready to take risks
4. I will always have a backup plan
5. I am creative
6. I'm a boss
7. I've got everything I need to be a successful person
8. I fear nothing
9. I am smart
10. I have a passion for whatever I do
11. I trust in my capabilities
12. My hard work will pay off.
13. I am blessed with unique talents.
14. My voice will be heard
15. I'm not going to give up
16. I can achieve anything without limits
17. I'm not going to doubt myself
18. My challenges make me stronger
19. I turn my failures into stepping stones
20. I own and am in control of my destiny.

21. I created my definition of success; I'm not pressured
22. I have ideas for success overflowing through me
23. Other people's expectations of me do not define my success
24. It is my time to succeed, and that I will do.
25. When hard times come, I go through them patiently.
26. I am proud of myself and what I have achieved
27. I make the best decisions to forge ahead
28. It's not more accessible, I get stronger and better
29. I'm not a failure; I learn and win.
30. I have the power to overcome my challenges.
31. I beat on every side.

KEY POINTS

1. An entrepreneur is responsible for the running of a venture or investing in an already established organization
2. Without passion for an experience, it will most likely fail.
3. There's much more to do apart from having the power, however
4. Entrepreneurship is for everyone.
5. Entrepreneurship is never easy.

CHAPTER TWELVE

SELF-LOVE

"You are what you believe yourself to be."
~Paulo Coelho

I think the concept of 'self-love' is something we're all too familiar with, yet it's not emphasized enough. Hence, I strive to explain what it means and how and why you should practice it as simply and concisely as I can. Chapter two of my book, "Milestones," with the title, "Self-love and The Black Woman," encompassed a lot about self-love and how to love yourself. It's a great book.

Honestly, you should read it sometime.

Before we go into the day's business, I've got a quick story to share, the story of my perfect friend, God rest her soul, and I believe it will help drive the point home about what self-love truly means.

Nancy was a promising young woman who was just about to clock twenty-seven and walk the altar with the man she had always loved all her life when we heard the news that she had committed suicide. It still hurts me today because I knew why, and when she told me about her problems, I had tried my best to make her want to relax from the negative thoughts, but I guess it wasn't enough.

Nancy always complained of being treated wrongly by her fiance, and at one point, it pissed me off because everyone was telling her to quit. He was too toxic, often gas lighting her and playing the manipulative card to the point that she had low-self-esteem, inferiority complex, and self-loathe. I had never seen anyone hate themself as much as Nancy did. Her fiancé, whose name I choose to withhold for? Reasons, made her believe she would never be good enough and that he was only doing her a favor being with her. He downplayed her intelligence and dished spiteful words at her daily.

"I'll never be good enough." Those were Nancy's last words to me before she died, and it shouldn't be a surprise why she said that. Amongst a host of other things, she was being bullied and manipulated adversely; I believe Nancy lacked self-love.

Self-love is a powerful force against people who wish to bring you down. Very powerful. Do you know how it is with those comical characters and their superpowers, like Batman, Superman, and Flash? Yeah, that's how self-love is with humans. It gives you this form of protection, like a coating against any negative thought, and here's an illustration.

Say, for example, you love yourself so much that you believe you can achieve anything you set your mind to, that nobody is allowed to talk down on you, and that you're the only one who can make or mar your life by the decisions you make, it would be hard for someone to come up at you and say you're a nobody. Go back to the quote by Paulo Coelho and reread it. Yes, my beautiful black woman, you are what you believe yourself to be. If you think you're beautiful, then you are. If you say, "Nah, that woman's way more beautiful than me. I've got such a big nose and acne spots all over my face and body, I'll never be able to compete with her," you've got it all wrong. First of all, you're not in a competition with anyone, this is all about you and yourself, and that is one point I need you to carry along as we talk correctly about what self-love means.

WHAT IS SELF-LOVE?

Self-love is a basis for all humans to thrive, and I'd like us to look past the negative aspects of it concerning vanity, pride, and selfishness because that's what comes to most people's minds nowadays. Some would say, "Oh, I love my body, I've got the smoothest skin in the world, and there's nothing anyone can do about it or say to hurt me anymore."

What would happen to you if misfortune comes your way and your skin becomes scalded? I'm not saying you don't love yourself, don't admire yourself. Heck, far from that. I'm saying self-love is beyond your physical attributes, so yes, you can try out all the facial and body care regimens, but within you, you're continuously thinking of how much of a failure you are, whipping yourself in the dark and wishing you had just enough courage to end it all. But what if I told you that it's not courage you lack but self-love? The American Association of Suicidology has stated that the risk of suicide is increased daily by the lack of self-love. So congratulate yourself because you've chosen to push through and not give in to self-loathe.

Remember that courage is the ability to remain strong in the face of adversity, so choosing to stay through it all and hoping for a better future is something brave of which I must commend you!

Self-love involves:

- Accepting yourself fully.
- Treat yourself with utmost kindness and respect.
- Nurturing your daily growth and wellbeing.

One must also be aware that self-love does not only embrace how you treat yourself but also how you think and feel about yourself. So, when you try to understand self-love, you would have to imagine what you would do for yourself, how you would talk to yourself about yourself, and how you would feel about yourself, reflecting love and concern for yourself.

Loving yourself gives you an overall positive view of yourself. It doesn't necessarily mean that you feel positive about yourself every single time; that's just crazy and would be unrealistic!

This is it; for example, there's nothing wrong with temporarily feeling upset, angry, or disappointed in yourself. It happens a lot to me, but that doesn't mean I hate myself. I still love myself, of course!

Don't let this confuse you; however, I'm here to put you through, so I'll ensure you get every bit of information right.

Just think about how things work in your relationships with other people. For example, I love my son even when I feel like locking him up in prison for a week. Even amid my anger and disappointment, my love for him will influence how I relate to him. It enables me to forgive him, look at things from his point of view, consider his feelings, meet his needs, and make decisions that will support his wellbeing. It is how self-love works. It is very much the same. And this means that if you know how to love others, you know how to love yourself! Or it's more like; if you know how to love yourself, you'd know how to love others.

SELF-LOVE VS NARCISSISM

Now, in addition to the fact that people question the necessity of self-love, another loophole in the practice of self-love is that people believe it's narcissistic or selfish. But that's not the case at all.

That's far from the truth, and I'm here to testify.

In encouraging self-love, psychologists and therapists do not mean anyone should put himself on a pedestal above everyone else. The thing with narcissists is that they believe that they're better than everyone else and will never concede or be responsible for their mistakes and flaws. They're also obsessed with seeking overwhelming amounts of validation and recognition from people. Narcissists also lack empathy for others.

On the contrary, self-love has nothing to do with showing off how much of a great person you are; that's just being delusional.

The people who love themselves in the best way are very much aware that they are flawed in their way and make mistakes, and they accept and care about themselves despite their imperfections. Self-love doesn't stop you from extending the arms of care to others; it just means that you can give yourself the same kindness you give to others.

PERFECTIONISM AND ILLS

The Ills of Perfectionism

Unfortunately, most of us in the Western world have been groomed to believe that the "quality" of perfectionism is a great one to have. After all, being overly obsessed with details leads to excellent work and perfect results. And this personality trait gives us something to brag about during job interviews.

Quality? Really? It's appalling that people think perfectionism is a quality or a virtue. But honestly, to me, it's a vice and one of the toxicity components. There's nothing good about perfectionism, nothing at all!

I want to re-emphasize that perfectionism is destructive for you (bad isn't the word). Not just "not ideal" or "harmful when excessive," but actively deficient in its ordinary sense, like doing drugs or being obese.

Now I'd like to let you know something. Are you aware that a shorter lifespan, irritable bowel syndrome, fibromyalgia, eating disorders, depression, and suicidal tendencies are only a few of the adverse health effects of perfectionism?

I don't think you thought it was that serious, but trust me, I don't even advise you to try because it may eat you up before you're aware and can come out of it, and that's a fact, my queen. There's no good side to this one.

Another revelation here; trying to recover from heart disease or cancer is also harder for people under the bandage of perfectionism, which makes the few who survive and the general populace more prone to anxiety and depression afterward.

DEALING WITH PERFECTIONISM

Now that we've established what perfectionism is all about, we don't have to waste too much time before we try to figure out what we can do to move away from perfectionism.

Well, first things first, you have to be humane enough to accept that it's not a good thing for you. Constantly berating yourself over every little error will slowly but surely chop away your sense of self-worth, making you a less happy person, and you need no one to let you know that you deserve better.

Like Kristin Neff, a human development professor at Texas University at Austin, said — "Love, connection, and acceptance are your birthright."

In essence, being happy is what you're entitled to, not something you need to earn or have someone give to you. Even the United Nations adopted a resolution recognizing that the "pursuit of happiness is a fundamental human goal." it's that important, my queens, don't ever let anyone or anything take that sense of self-worth from you. Not your boss, not your friends, not your ex!

Again, you should also try your very best to resist the urge to beat yourself up for beating yourself. Sounds strange? It shouldn't. In simpler terms, you don't need to kill yourself for being a perfectionist in trying to break out from the shackles of perfectionism. That's just doing what you're trying your best not to.

And if you think you're doing yourself a favor, I'm afraid you're only making things worse.

According to Paul Hewitt, a clinical psychologist in Vancouver, Canada, and author of the book *"Perfectionism: A Relational Approach to Conceptualization, Assessment, and Treatment,"* the inner critic harbored by perfectionists could be the same as *"a nasty adult beating the crap out of a tiny child."*

You'd probably see something like that in reality and be like *"Damn, what sort of monster does that to a child?"*

But then you're unaware that you do that to yourself daily. How ironic. You need to look inward, ladies.

Spending many years grooming this inner bully, you develop an unconscious reflex to always bring yourself down for every minor thing, no matter how ridiculous.

You know, the little things can drive you crazy, from missing a deadline by even just a day to dropping a teaspoon on the floor; one thing is sure, perfectionists will constantly award themselves a hard time over the most unexpected things, so I don't think criticizing yourself for criticizing yourself is very rare. It happens, man, it happens.

Then again, it's possible to start working towards some much-needed self-compassion. You might feel like self-love is a case of *"you either have it, or you don't,"* but the good news is that psychologists have insisted that it is something you can learn.

So you see, there's hope! Don't give up on yourself, because the moment you do, you give up on everything else!

WHY PRACTICE SELF-LOVE?

It's pretty glaring, ladies; if you don't love yourself, who else will you, love? I mean, it's humanly impossible to love others if you don't love yourself. I don't mean to be too harsh when I say that you're going to be a nuisance to whoever you come across or try to have a relationship with if you don't love yourself enough.

That's the central truth because you will think you're trying your best to love, but you discover that it isn't just working out no matter how hard you try.

And then you begin to feel like everyone hates you, but you don't even know why?

There isn't much to talk about the need for self-love. It's glaring!

It's your right to be happy! There are no "10 reasons why you need to love yourself" this is just it right here, ladies; it is a necessity for healthy living.

You've got to wake up every day and always choose to love yourself no matter what!

And that's on, period, ladies!

HOW DO YOU PRACTICE SELF-LOVE?

Quit The Comparisons

I don't think anyone would boldly say that they haven't found themselves comparing themselves with other people. It happens, but you have to stop making it an everyday thing.

Making comparisons is too toxic to do every day because you take the worst parts of your life and compare them to the best interests of someone else. And you're willing to do that to yourself often so much that you make it a habit?

Think again, dear. Think again.

Be Around People You Feel Good With

If you're constantly surrounding yourself with people who make you feel less of yourself, you might want to change your circle for the good of your mental health.

You can't be around people who make you feel good, and then you won't tap from some of that energy, and you can't surround yourself with people who make you think you shouldn't exist and not be affected by their negativity. That's how it works. Jim Rohn said:

"You are the ordinary five people you spend the most time with."

Think about who those people currently are. Do they inspire you and want what's best for you?

Worry Less

If you don't know by now, worry accentuates self-hate.

I'm going to use this example; you took an examination and didn't do well when the results were out. The average human reaction is to feel bad about the situation and then begin to worry. Letting that feeling linger for longer than usual may not be too good for your mental health because when you begin to worry too much about the results, you start beating yourself up for not being up to standard or for not being intelligent enough to pass the exams and that's a breeding ground for self-hate if you'd ask me.

Quit worrying; it doesn't solve any problem.

There's this thing about the worry I learned.

Why are you worried? Is it something that can be done? Please do it!

Is it otherwise?

Then why worry?

Why?

Go Easy on Yourself

You know, sometimes, when you need to love yourself the most, you end up treating yourself like you shouldn't exist. And that's putting salt on the injury. I find it appalling that some people see such a thing as therapeutic. Well, I don't! Some people call it motivation, but to be honest, you're just being crazy if you do that.

I'm not saying that you should strive for self-improvement or not accept that you've done wrong or something of that sort, but after that moment of chastising yourself for a mistake, brace up!

The world isn't waiting for you to finish telling yourself how stupid you are before it continues moving; it doesn't care about you; the only person that can genuinely care about you is you! So why do otherwise?

Go easy on yourself, woman, everyone makes mistakes, and we're expected to learn from them and not sulk over them for eternity.

Make Room for Healthy Habits

I want to ask you all a question.

How do you feel after doing some form of workout, say, jogging around your neighborhood a couple of times?

Well, I don't know about you, but I feel perfect about myself when I do stuff like that. Even when I'm tired, that good feeling overshadows that tiredness to a great extent.

Do you know why? I'll tell you why I think I feel good.

Everyone knows that working out keeps the body healthy, strong, and fit.

Working out makes me feel like I'm taking a step in the right direction to put my health in order, making me feel on top of the world!

I'd be like, yeah, something's going to feel good in my body in a couple of months or years, and that's one of the things that excite me a lot.

Even when it comes as a dare, maybe I was dared by a friend to do twenty or fifty push-ups. When I complete the task, it makes me feel accomplished, and for a moment, I feel like I can take on anything life throws at me.

You don't get that feeling often as an adult, so whatever you need to do to get it, I advise you to do it.

AFFIRMATIONS

1. I love myself
2. I allow myself to heal
3. I'm OK with moving at my own pace
4. I'm grateful for wherever I am in life right now
5. I'm looking forward to the best that is yet to come
6. I'm at peace with myself
7. I will forgive myself
8. I get better every day
9. The world needs me
10. I will always prioritize taking care of myself
11. I deserve everything I dream of.
12. Good things are coming to me
13. I do not feel insecure about myself
14. I am wanted
15. I am strong

16. I am working on being the best version of myself every day
17. What people have to say about me doesn't affect me
18. I will never give up on myself when life gets hard
19. Everything is going to work out for me
20. I will always be kind to myself.
21. I am letting go of whatever I'm worried about.
22. Some things can't change, and I am OK with that.
23. I am in total harmony and balance with life
24. I am learning how to be supportive of my best self
25. All is well in my world; I am calm, happy, and content
26. I will make time for myself every day because I am worth it.
27. I will always appreciate myself and find other things to be grateful for
28. I'm going to stop beating up myself; it doesn't help me
29. I will not be held back by the weight of my regrets
30. I try my best at all times.
31. All my efforts bring good results.
32. I am full of love.

KEY POINTS

1. It's impossible not to love yourself and love others
2. Self-love is different from Narcissism
3. Self-love can be learned
4. Nobody is perfect
5. Mental struggles always have a way of affecting your physical health.

CHAPTER THIRTEEN

MENTAL/EMOTIONAL HEALING

"There is a crack in everything, that's how the light gets in."
- Leonard Cohen

Anyone able to read this has, in one way or the other, been mentally and emotionally hurt. Even the most muscular man on earth has been emotionally hurt before.

Come on! You know how stuff like this works, don't you? And I fear that if I start to give examples, it might trigger past sad memories. So I'm just going to assume that you know what I'm talking about and hope my assumption is correct.

However, we're not dwelling too much on the pain but the healing because that's the only way you'll move forward in life. Well yeah.

So let's move on to what we have next.

WHAT IS EMOTIONAL HEALING?

First, you must know that emotional healing is not a one-day thing but a process; it is a process of accepting all the hurtful experiences that life has brought your way and whatever adverse emotional reaction such experiences have triggered. It means mastering the art of coping with the numerous darts thrown our way in the course of living.

It indeed doesn't materialize in a day or two, but when one is emotionally healed, the mental pain which makes life a little bit unbearable to live (as the case may be) does not hold someone back; to a considerable extent, the mental wounds are closed, and there is no significant pain.

And I speak for all of you when I say that the joy of getting over an emotional trauma is second to none. It's like you've been given a second chance at life after being dead for some time. That feeling of relief is undoubtedly worth the number of times you had to cry to bed, skip meals and classes, and shut yourself from the outside world.

WHY EMOTIONAL HEALING?

Is this even supposed to be a question? It amuses me sometimes why one must stress why emotional healing is necessary.

I mean, rather than someone living the rest of his days in the anguish of mental distraught, why not heal and get it over with? It's much better, ladies, or don't you think so? Well, if you don't, I honestly do think so regardless, and I'd wish for you to have a rethink too.

Mental healing teaches us a lot of life lessons on how to cope and adjust to certain life issues. It gives you an insight into emotional reactions resulting from these life struggles, which will, in turn, help you express your feelings in the best way possible.

When you think carefully before acting upon a situation, it'll save you a lot of stress, and you may not even be aware of it.

That's one truth I'll always stand by. That decision you took after thinking critically, even if it might not have gone the exact way you wanted it, would've been worse if you took another impulse decision.

Finding purpose and meaning connects well with others, and then focusing on good things in life happens. And that's as a result of mental healing. It opens your eyes to many things you may have missed while grieving.

EFFECTS OF EMOTIONAL PAIN

Mental hurt is never easy to conceal. There are no physical injuries, broken bones, or spilled blood, but whatever is going on within your broken heart will always find a way to show itself; most times, you wouldn't notice until you sit and think or someone draws it to attention.

These are some of the reactions of a broken heart that needs healing.

Anger

Most of the time, the people who have nothing to do with whatever pain you're facing are the people who are at the receiving end of your anger. Your very close friends, family, or even a passerby could have a taste of that bitterness caused by your ex, maybe, or your boss and co-workers.

And then even people on the Internet who you've never met or seen by accident before! I know a lot of things like this, especially on Twitter.

A person could be sharing their opinion about something on the net, and then someone comes up with a highly bizarre comment that leaves everyone wondering if everything is fine at home.

Yeah, that person could need healing, you know?

Low Self-Esteem

You might often feel like you're not enough (we're going to be looking at this next, so stay tuned.)

It could be two things. Maybe you faulted, maybe did something to offend a friend, and then whenever you remember what you did, you feel guilt, shame, and disbelief in yourself. That's a tough nut to crack, to be honest, when you're wrong.

But the other case could be you being manipulated into thinking that you're the wrong person. Most issues arise from toxic relationships where the guy always wants to make his girl feel like she's the cause of every one of the fights they have and may even push her to break up with him and then blame her for ruining the relationship.

These are two different scenarios, but they trigger the same feeling, and it's hard to let go of guilt sometimes.

Holding Onto Grudges

People who are emotionally damaged find it hard to forgive. And while you may think that's evil behavior to have as a human being, you may never really understand why they're like that or how they turned out that way. Some people have been hurt by people they thought would never hurt them, and that's enough to drive you crazy, man!

It makes it hard for them not to trust or believe in what they say. It's a toxic way of life, but to them, it's their security, so I don't even want to have a say about why they turned out to be like that.

Insomnia

We can't rule out the physical effects of being heartbroken. Even apart from being unable to find sleep, you feel physically tired most of the time because you've been overthinking lately, and it's wearing you up and tearing you apart.

You didn't have a siesta, so why are you finding it hard to go to bed at night? There are so many ways a human can be tortured, but then the deprivation of sleep comes close to the top. One thing again is that you're not even being productive while you're awake. How can you be effective when you can't even think straight?

Sometimes, there could be a particular thing in your mind, maybe the incident where you have hurt, and then again, there could be absolutely nothing in your mind; you're just staring into the blank space with an empty mind, listening to sad songs to heighten the pain.

Imagine being in so much pain that you want to feel it, probably to know what more it can do to you.

That's quite sad; I wouldn't wish that on anyone; that's a horrible way to live.

STAGES OF HEALING

I've said this before, but I'd like to repeat that no human life is free from challenges or crises. The earlier we understand this, the better.

Yeah, no one wants to experience hardships in their lives, but we have to understand that a crisis is a state that initiates a turning point in our lives. Since we cannot avoid it, we must know how to survive and understand the emotional stages we go through to bounce back from dramatic life changes.

I mentioned a few reactions we might have when we're going through trauma. These feelings form part of the healing or adjustment process, which is long and different for each individual.

A person goes through five stages as they shuffle through the healing process. It is important to note that these stages last for different periods and replace each other, or at times coexist and are not the same for every individual.

STAGE ONE: GRIEF AND DENIAL

We all know what grief is, don't we? Well, it is intense mental suffering caused by specific life issues, like the loss of a relationship, loss of a loved one, loss of a job, and so many more we all know.

I'm telling you the truth, no matter how toxic your relationship was with your ex, a sense of loss still exists when you end things. Memories you don't want to let replay in your head, and the thought that you wouldn't be able to get them again makes you sad.

Anyway, before accepting your loss, there's a tendency that you will deny it, and that tendency is very high, I tell you.

You're going to think to yourself,

"I refuse to believe this is happening to me!"

Denial is quite the norm. Humans use it as a defense against painful emotional experiences that they have difficulty stopping.

However, slowly but surely, you will look at your loss and accept it with faith and growing optimism for a better future.

STAGE TWO: ANGER

Anger is what usually follows after the grief and denial stage. This is the stage where we ask whoever is listening why we have to go through what we go through.

Sometimes you might even be surprised at how angry you are about whatever situation got you into a mess and why it had to happen.

For instance, you broke up with your boyfriend some days ago because he cheated on you. You're going to notice that you might be asking yourself specific questions at a point in your life.

"Why did he have to cheat?"

"Why didn't he tell me he wasn't interested in me?"

These questions are expressions of your anger. Sometimes you know it hasn't happened like that, but that's how life chose to happen, and we can't do anything about it.

However, recognizing anger helps you move on to the next stage, which matters.

STAGE THREE: BARGAINING

This is usually a call for a retrace. After dealing with anger for some time, you may want to return to your toxic boss who just served you a sack letter thinking that if you act or talk nicely or "bargains," decisions may be reversed, and you might have a second shot at the job.

For example, you might say, *"I promise I won't rebel against you if you give me another chance at the office."*

While doing that, you're still hoping that things change for the better and your boss stops being a toxic one. But what's the assurance that such will ever happen? That's why I prefer that you let go. But then, it's something we might have to go through as we go through the healing process.

STAGE FOUR: DEPRESSION

This stage is the deadliest of all stages in the healing process. Severe depression could lead to worse irreversible situations like suicide, and once one has been able to come out of this situation, nothing can hold the person back.

You know we talked about anger the other time. That type of anger was easily expressed and was usually directed at the other party causing you the pain.

This time, depression usually takes the form of unexpressed anger turned inward on yourself. At this point, you think you can no longer do anything to make yourself feel better. (This is usually where suicidal tendencies creep in)

Depression also comes with you losing your sense of self-worth. In truth, this is the most challenging stage and makes one feel withdrawn, exhausted, and helpless. You might not be aware, but that feeling of helplessness hits so complexly and differently. Like, you can't do anything to fix your life; that's one of the worst feelings to have as a human being.

By expression, passive anger is transformed into active anger, which allows us to see things objectively. Depression, however, makes this very hard to achieve.

STAGE FIVE: ACCEPTANCE

It sounds like it, but acceptance is not a happy stage. It is a stage characterized by a feeling of emptiness, as if the pain is gone, the struggle is over, and rest is at hand. At this stage, faith begins to strengthen, and growth follows. Then a new life is within your reach. This is positive about this stage and not even happiness.

A crisis can do a lot for many people, and people fail to realize this. It can be a person's force to break old habits and bring about unprecedented change. Don't try to rush the process; you must allow time to bring healing, and above all, you must be willing to be a healed person.

While healing, identify your own emotional needs and set realistic goals. Where do you want to be a month from now or a year from now?

These are the five stages of healing. While you go through these stages, you're not aware of the progress, and the realization usually hits when you've healed completely.

Then you can reminisce and pinpoint the various stages of your healing. You'd only look back and smile at them because you've gone through a lot, and you deserve whatever freedom and happiness come after passing through the excruciating pain of healing.

POSITIVE AFFIRMATIONS FOR MENTAL HEALING

1. I'm going to use whatever hurdle life brings my way to be a better person
2. I am willing to forgive myself
3. I accept and learn from the lessons my pain is teaching me
4. I believe that everything in my life is unfolding the way it should
5. I will be kind to myself
6. I am willing to amend whatever lousy behavior I have
7. As I forgive myself, I am ready to forgive others
8. Everything I'm going through is making me stronger, wiser, and a better person overall
9. The love I expect from others, I'm willing to give back
10. I will always permit myself to heal
11. I am responsible for the quality of my relationships
12. Weeping may endure for a night, but joy comes in the morning
13. I will always allow genuine love into my life and be willing to give as well
14. I acknowledge the past and look forward to a better future
15. My body knows how to heal itself, and I won't interrupt its healing process.
16. My past defines my present and future
17. I am aware of the signals my feelings give to me, and I acknowledge them
18. I am letting go of the past; I chose to live now and in the moment
19. I am thriving in my healing journey
20. I see every new day as a day full of hope and happiness.
21. I let go of the past and believe that everything is working for my good
22. I wish myself well every single day
23. I am open to new ways of healing myself
24. I'm at peace with my body, heart, mind, and soul

25. Happy thoughts play a significant role in my healing process
26. Perfect health is a divine right, and I'm claiming it now
27. I let go of any impediments to my perfect healing
28. Every bridge I need to burn, I do so to better my mental health
29. I'm allowed to have evil days. I am human
30. I experience happiness every day.
31. My grief does not engulf me.
32. I forgive myself for all the times I took part in creating my grief.
33. I will come out of my hurt stronger and happier.
34. I have all it takes to heal.
35. I curate my joys.
36. My pain will not last forever.

KEY POINTS

1. The healing process is not a one-day thing
2. Healing without learning will only leave the wounds open
3. The healing stages do not always coincide. Sometimes they even coexist
4. No human has not experienced a crisis
5. A crisis is a state that initiates a turning point in our lives.

CHAPTER FOURTEEN

YOU ARE ENOUGH

"Know your worth! People always act like they're doing more for you than you're doing for them."

-Kanye West

Having spoken to you about so many aspects of your lives, how things work around them, how to make improvements, and the sort, what's a better way to end the whole thing than letting you know you're enough?

No one is perfect, and everyone has their weak points; your toxic partner that always seeks perfection from you is also hopelessly flawed.

There are a few things concerning your behavior that you might want to put in place because of the ones you love, and that's fine; making efforts to improve is always a wonderful sight to behold, but you ought to know when to stop struggling and accept yourself the way that you've come to be because everyone makes mistakes and the people who you love, that you're trying to make adjustments for, if they don't recognize your efforts, then I firmly believe that they're not worth loving. You should focus your energy on loving the people that do appreciate you and will accept and love you for the person that you are.

This topic can be viewed from many angles, but we will be looking at it from the tip of our self-worth this time. In other words, we will focus on your self-worth and your recognition of self-worth. A lot of misfortunes in the life of people are birthed by the lack of recognition of their self-worth.

For example, a lady will choose to stay in a toxic relationship because her toxic partner always wants to make her believe that she's nothing without him and that he's the only flavor or color in her life. Because she doesn't realize that she's important, these words and actions get to her; she believes him and stays with him, enduring all the pain and anguish that comes as a result of being in a toxic relationship, and in the end, it leaves her feeling damaged beyond repair. (She feels damaged beyond repair even if there's always hope for the living to be whole).

It could lead to depression, and then there's a possibility that she wouldn't be able to take it anymore and may decide to take matters into her own hands and end things.

That's quite unfortunate—a sad ending to a probably once happy life because one didn't recognize her self-worth.

One thing I always pray for as I pen these words down is that as you take a good look at this book, you can take something to run with. That'll be my greatest joy, honestly. Know that many people are gaining value from whatever I have to offer.

So let's begin. Where do we start?

WHAT IS SELF-WORTH?

Before we define self-worth, we must understand the relationship between self-esteem and self-worth. If you think they're the same. I'm here to tell you they're not, and I will tell you why.

Self-esteem is what we think, feel and believe about ourselves and then self-worth is recognizing that you're bigger than all of those things.

Don't understand yet? Leave that to me; I'd do the explaining.

As humans, there are many things we feel about ourselves, good or bad. For example, you may realize that you're always a little too tardy anywhere you go. To class, place of work, church, or any special event you've been to. Now you're not denying that you're a person who doesn't keep to time; that's not what self-worth means. You recognize that you're a delinquent, but don't allow it to bring you down anytime you think about it. You believe that you can overcome it as well! That's self-worth in a nutshell, acknowledging that you're not perfect but not allowing your imperfections to get the better of you.

THE NEED FOR SELF-WORTH

Self-worth is a beautiful thing to have. Many benefits are associated with feeling good about yourself and not allowing your imperfections to drag you back.

We're going to discuss a few benefits of having self-worth, and I hope you find a reason to build on your self-worth if you haven't started before now.

Confident Approach to Solving Problems

Lack of self-worth leaves you feeling like you can't come up with some idea that could be helpful to solve specific problems you may come across in life.

Even if you come up with a good idea, you'd always feel like it's not good enough and won't amount to something substantial. You know what's worse, even when you've got some sort of approval from others, you still feel that there's this missing piece you're looking to fill and that you'd never be able to fill it in.

However, when your sense of self-worth is intact, you will feel confident when making decisions. Because you believe in yourself to work out solutions for yourself, things will turn out great! Even if things don't turn out as you expected, you're still not discouraged because you're willing to learn from your mistakes and try some other time again, feeling more confident to do the right thing.

Realistic Expectations

You may think that when I say someone has a sense of self-worth, I mean that such a person thinks they are perfect and can do no wrong. Well, that's not how it works. It's the other way round.

People who value themselves are not so keen on perfection. They do not demand perfection from themselves.

The reason is that the connection with their essential humanity is so intact that they know it isn't a realistic goal for themselves or others to want to be perfect. And as a result, they don't feel threatened or pressured by the fact that they and others will make mistakes or that the world they live in isn't always safe and reliable.

Have Healthier Relationships

You're going to have a more honest and healthier relationship with people when your sense of self-worth is considerably high, and this is because you don't ever feel the need to hide who you are. You know, many people always look to impress, and as a result, they go the extra mile to pretend and hide the kind of person they are because they believe they're not going to be accepted if they show their true selves.

That wouldn't be the case for a person with a sense of self-worth. Such a person would prefer to be known for who he is than pretend to be someone else to get approval that may not add anything to their lives. We all know that a relationship founded on false characters won't last long and wouldn't even be healthy while it lasts.

It goes for romantic and working relationships, friendships, and family relationships. They'd become more honest and healthier when their self-worth is intact.

Resilience

Many people think that you become immune to setbacks when you value yourself. However, that's not the case at all. Instead, a sense of self-worth makes you more resilient to setbacks; that's the word. Resilience!

When you don't think highly of yourself, the tendency to feel devastated by failures and losses is very high, and those losses may take their toll on you even if they're relatively minor. You may begin to see them as signs that you are a terrible person or a loser.

But things are different when you feel good about yourself; you're never going to feel like an irredeemable failure even after something you've done didn't go as it should. You're not blind to the knowledge that you've failed, but you don't generalize that label to include your identity. You have to deal with bad things and move on when bad things happen to you.

These are a few benefits of valuing yourself, and everyone is valid.

Everyone wants to be confident in making decisions concerning solving problems; nobody wants to feel bad because they're not perfect; being in a healthy relationship is a goal for many people, and indeed, no one wants to feel like a failure because of one setback they had.

If no one told you before, I'm here to tell you that building your self-worth is a game changer and would quickly make the above needs within reach.

HOW TO IMPROVE YOUR SELF-WORTH

Having spoken a bit on the benefits of having a high sense of self-worth, it'll only be fair to discuss how to overcome low self-esteem and develop high self-esteem to become a better person.

There are a lot and a lot of them, but I'm only going to discuss a few with you.

If you're struggling with a low sense of self-worth, I hope you check them out, and trust me, when you put them into practice, there's going to be a difference, and you're going to notice how better life will begin to look.

Identify and Confront your Negative Beliefs

You're losing your sense of self-worth because these negative beliefs are all over your head. You have to notice those thoughts and challenge them as soon as possible.

For example, you might notice yourself having thoughts like:

"I'm not smart enough to pass this test"

"I'll never be good enough for this relationship."

"I've got no friends."

And so many more negative thoughts are constantly ringing in your head.

However, when you notice these thought patterns, look for evidence that contradicts those statements. Then proceed to write down both comments and evidence. Do well to keep looking back at what you've written down to remind yourself that your negative beliefs about yourself are false.

Come to Terms with the Positives

It is just like doing the opposite of what I spoke about earlier. This time, you're affirming the good things you notice about yourself, which is an excellent way to start.

You can also write down those things that you're good at and things that have earned you external compliments and affection. When you start to feel low, look back on those things you've written to remind yourself that there's still a lot of good in you.

When you start, don't write yourself off when falling back to the old negative habits because they're all part of the process. But with consistent effort, you will find yourself doing better with time and building your self-esteem.

Do What You Love

When you do what you love and are passionate about, there's this eternal urge to want to get better by all means possible, and even when you fail at it, you're optimistic that one day you'll get better, so you don't beat yourself up. Instead, you keep on trying to get better.

Well, if it is the other way round, you'd hardly find fulfillment in whatever you do. And when you fail at it, it becomes a bigger problem because you're not so willing to improve, which bullies you into thinking you'll never get better at it.

Even though you can get better at doing things you don't like, why not do what you want and rest easy knowing that you're going after your passion?

Receive Compliments

People think they're being modest when someone compliments them, and they're like:

"Oh! Can you stop? See. I didn't even hit that pitch aesthetically, or I didn't get the painting completely right, or I didn't score as many goals as I should've."

I used to think that way, too, until I understood that it wasn't doing me any good.

When someone compliments your work, you need to stop looking at that work from your perspective; instead, look at that work from the eyes of the person who has complimented you. Please focus on the things they've said you did well in particular and appreciate yourself for that because you can't always be perfect, so there's no need to try to chase it.

So accept the compliments you receive and move with the satisfaction you've impressed someone in your heart.

Address Yourself With Care

You've got to be careful of how you address yourself so that you don't damage your sense of self-worth by speaking, so I'll tell you that you become what you've said.

You can do this by checking how you use the expression *"I am."*

The expression is strong, and you've got to be careful how you use it. Most of the time, some people react to a mistake they've made by insulting themselves.

"Oh! I am such a fool."
"Oh damn! I'm so stupid for trying to do that."

But is that who they are? Not!

Some people say that it makes them feel good when they insult themselves, but I think that's just being delusional. There is no such thing as that; I refuse to believe it!

If at all you should talk down on yourself after making a mistake, you should approach things a different way. Why not talk down on the action or thought rather than yourself? That's a much better way to approach things rather than call yourself names you do not bear.

You could say,

"I didn't do that thing right." Or

"That idea wasn't a good one."

You know, it kind of moves you out of the ridicule and places what your actions were instead.

The whole idea is that you're not what you've done, so there isn't a need to talk down on yourself. Talk down on the mistake instead; it's healthier.

I wish I could go further, but this will be all.

These are just a few, and I hope you all try them and also not be too hard on yourself when you don't get it right sometimes.

POSITIVE AFFIRMATIONS

1. I am enough
2. I don't need to change; I can only get better.
3. No matter how small, I contribute my quota to the world
4. I love myself more and more each passing day
5. I am unique, and I don't need to be someone I'm not for anyone to like me
6. I am talented, creative, and full of crazy ideas.
7. I have confidence in the decisions I make
8. I will not give up on myself.
9. There's good in me, and I will focus on that and not the bad I tend to see in myself
10. I am my best friend
11. I am beautiful regardless of what others have to say about me
12. I believe I have a bright future
13. I will be careful with the words I say about myself
14. I am grateful for who I am
15. I see myself through kind eyes
16. I will not criticize myself before others do
17. I can face every challenge
18. I don't need external validation to know my worth

19. I am in complete control of my emotions
20. I'm thankful for this journey so far
21. I have the power to create everything I want in life
22. I know what I'm worth and will not lessen myself for anyone else
23. I am one of a kind; there is no one like me
24. My existence makes the world a better place
25. I can find whatever I am looking for within me
26. I am worthy of being praised and rewarded for my efforts
27. I am stronger than my struggles
28. I constantly bask in pure and positive energy
29. I am the only one who can determine my self-worth
30. I'm worth it.
31. I trust my ideas and potential.
32. I am the queen of my life.
33. I am enough at every point.

KEY POINTS

1. Self-worth places you above what you think about yourself
2. Perfection is a myth
3. We can't always get it right
4. Self-worth builds confidence
5. There will always be a chance to do better.

Conclusion

Dear black woman! Congratulations on getting to the last page of this book.

I hope these affirmations pull you out of your dark days, I hope you feel happy saying them aloud to yourself too. Always remember that it is what you declare that you become. Now, go all out and be badass and tell yourself the sweetest things while at it.

I love you.

Thank You

You could have picked from dozens of other books, but you picked our bundle of 2 books

Feminine Affirmations for Black Women

So, THANK YOU for getting this book and for making it all the way to the end.

Could you please consider posting a review on Amazon or if you get the Audio version then on Audible?

Posting a positive review is the best and easiest way to support the work of independent authors like me.

Your feedback will help me to keep writing the kind of books that will help you get the results you want.

It can be something short and simple ☺

Spiritual Self-Care for Black Women:

Powerful Guide & Workbook to Help you Transform Your Life in 12 Months. Find Inner Peace, Happiness and Become Unstoppable. Develop Positive Mindset with Affirmations.

Introduction	**9**
CHAPTER ONE: IT'S NOT A COINCIDENCE!	17
CHAPTER TWO: KNOW YOURSELF!	29
CHAPTER THREE: IT'S ALL IN YOUR HANDS	40
CHAPTER FOUR: BUILDING UP YOUR SPIRITUAL ENERGY	48
CHAPTER FIVE: LIVING YOUR SPIRITUALITY	61
CHAPTER SIX	75
CHAPTER SEVEN: WHAT'S THE CONNECTION?	92

Twelve Months Transformation Journal: 135

Introduction

Spirituality is a brave search for the truth about existence, fearlessly peering into the mysterious nature of life.

—Elizabeth Lesser

When people hear "spirituality," they think of churches, mosques, temples, and shrines. But, spirituality is way beyond that. It is beyond religion and what the fanatics tell you. Spirituality is a journey to self and the powers and forces beyond self. I embarked on a personal mission to discover what spirituality means in my quest for knowledge. There is nothing as exciting as discovering meanings and unraveling them yourself.

Go back to the quote in the beginning. This time, read it slowly and carefully. There is one thing I want you to note, and that is a mystery. Many people fail to realize that life and human existence aren't all black and white as some people may make it seem. You aren't just dreams; you did not meet that stranger who became your best friend by chance. You did not become like that by mere coincidence. At the core of it all, a connecting force binds everything together. That force compounds our understanding; that is what makes mystery. Interesting, right? You'll find out more as I go further. I do not want to rush through this book like it is my favorite meal. For you, I'll take my time to go through every concept, belief, and curiosity delicately. This book is an opening from myself to you.

Before I proceed, there is something I need you to know. It answers a popular question that I have heard people ask. 'What is the best form of spirituality?' Even though I believe significantly in my ideology of spirituality, I do not consider it the best form of spirituality. Do you know why? It is because spirituality is a thing people experience on different levels. There are no two individuals that share the spiritual in the same ways. It is a personal thing. If you say your spirituality is the best, it's illogical because you would only be trying to compare two mutually exclusive things. That's not the way it works.

Fanatics and shallow people who do not even have firm standings on their spirituality are born in such unnecessary comparisons. I love to make things easy for people, especially for gorgeous black women like you, who I understand and love with the most significant portion of my heart. But this journey into the deep and the spiritual is one that I can't make easy for you. You have to experience it to know it, honestly.

No matter the tastiness of the pudding and the sharpness of my tongue, it is impossible for me to transfer the sweetness to your tongue. It is for you to do. That is why I urge you to seek spirituality by yourself. Do not give anyone the chance of filling you with fallacies.

I write this book for and to you with all the love I know, my dear black woman. You may never really find fulfillment without understanding this salient aspect of human life for yourself. Sadly, the subject is not given enough attention as it should. Right now, we're all about the money, the fame, the spotlights, and whatever we choose to be after, and we forget ourselves in the process. Don't you think that's a little bit absurd? I mean, it's pretty funny that we want all these for ourselves, and we're thinking, *"Oh, when I get these, I'm gonna live the life I want to live, I'm going to be satisfied, fulfilled."* And you know, all the thoughts that come with daydreaming about our future often don't go as planned or as dreamt.

But then I'll tell you that if it so happens that you got all that you wanted, whether, by luck or hard work, all that self-discovery, spirituality, and all that you left behind, chasing wealth and fame will still be there where you left it. Are you going to pay for therapy? That's a good idea. But then I hope you're not so broken that nothing can fix you by then. No doubt, treatment is good, very quintessential, in fact, in your journey to harness the full benefits of being able to understand your spirituality. Still, it's too much of a risk neglecting that part of your life because you're too busy hustling for what you want. Spirituality is what you need, an absolute necessity.

There's a guy I know that tries to be rational about everything. Everyone says he's a "cool" guy, and yeah, I think most people that think like him and always want to see things the way they are, are tagged "cool." But then this guy would meet a new person, and afterward, he'd be like, "I don't think my frequency resonates with that guy's," or he'd talk about how immediately comfortable he becomes while speaking to someone else. On a good day, I'd like to ask him his rationale for such emotions and how he already feels something about someone he doesn't know. No matter how we try to look at life from a neutral point of view, there's always something that happens that points beyond what we see. The earlier we understand our link to the spiritual manner and how to strike a balance, the better!

Earlier spoken, we must learn to separate spirituality from religion. No matter how similar these two concepts may seem, they're nowhere related. And please don't get me wrong here, ladies, love God, love Jesus, love Allah, love Buddha, the list goes on. Still, you have to make sure that while you love your religions and what they stand for, you don't forget to love yourself and do whatever it takes to get in touch with your spirituality because that's where self-care is born from. When you understand your spirituality, you will realize many things you need to do and things not to do, people you should avoid and people you shouldn't, places to be and places not to. Spirituality will open your eyes to a whole new side to life, and your perception will change for the better. You will also realize that there are boundaries that you need to set to make living easy. There's a lot of energy you don't need. You probably want it, but you don't need it. It's eating you up from the inside, and you're not aware of it, or maybe you enjoy being sad and depressed? But I highly doubt that. I mean, isn't that why you're here? Black woman, what if I tell you that you can free yourselves from that toxic cycle you cry through every day? If there were a way I could start this campaign for infant black girls, I would go the extra length to do that. But I guess not, so let's allow them to learn the alphabet letters till we can set the ball rolling for the young ones.

There's so much going on right now, and in one way or the other, they find a way to affect our lives whether we like it. With everything going on, why do we have to be a burden and let too much noise in when we know we can be free? It's a sacrifice that's worth it a hundred times over. Change begins with the individual; the change we seek to see in the world starts with us all; kind of cliché, but it drives home the point. When you understand your spirituality, you become better for yourself and others. When you're put in positions of power, the effect radiates, and your subordinates see this, and they'll come asking you.

"You seem really at ease with life; what's the secret?"

And then you'd flash a self-satisfied smile and reply to them.

"I embraced my spirituality, and you should embrace yours too."

Believe me; it works like magic when you're deep in it. You're changing the world from your corner and spreading the light. No matter how ridiculous it may sound, the world will be a better place when every one of us embraces our spirituality.

Why am I so confident about this? You're probably asking, or aren't you? Why is this writer so optimistic about this formula? Can one learn how to live? Well, we can't. We live and learn, make mistakes and move on, hoping that we don't make the same mistakes.

And one of the things we must learn as we live is how to understand our spirituality. If you're familiar with Grant Cardone's "Be Obsessed or Be Average," you'll know how he emphasized and re-emphasized the need to be obsessed. That's exactly how I will underline the need to understand your spirituality throughout this book. You'll see the word "spirituality" a lot in this book, and it's not because I don't know how to write a book. Nah, that's a far cry. It's the emphasis! I want you to see it over and over again till it sticks! It's just as important as regular exercise, healthy foods, and making money; it's the key to living life! And yeah, I'm so confident about it because It has worked for me. I wouldn't make a big deal about it if I didn't see the results. So yeah, understanding my spirituality has helped me in so many ways I can't even imagine. I will share some testimonies as we progress to let you see how this gospel can turn everything around.

It's not easy adjusting; it's not easy trying to get in touch with that spiritual side; it's not a piece of cake trying to embrace what you cannot see. But then, does anything come easy? The steps may be easy, but what exactly isn't easy is for you to begin following those steps. You may have resigned to fate and said;

"Damn it, whatever happens, happens anyway, so I'll just let life take its course." And then you stumbled upon this book, and you're like;

"This is my last shot, and if this doesn't work, then it's over."

In this introductory part of the book, I'd just let you know that you have a start! And be consistent! This book is not a spell. Even a bit requires you to move a wand. So this is me urging you to put in the work. This formula is a potent one, and it requires that you take action. Be intentional. Yes! It's not going to work itself out. It's a practical body of work, so it will be useless if you don't put it in the position. I'll be frank with you, I've put in so much work to put this together and get it across. So please make this work for my sake and yours. You're the most muscular woman I know. And I trust that you're going to kill this just like you're killing it in every other aspect of your life. You are the best mother, the best daughter, the best sister, and the best at living!

So as I draw the curtains to this introduction close, I need you to do something for me.

Place your hands on your chest and say these affirmations after me. Are you ready? Good.

"I, the most muscular woman in the world, aggressively swear to make the ride worthwhile. No pressure, slow, steady, till I get in touch with my spirituality and be even more potent than I thought.

So help me, God."

Now buckle your seat belts. I'll get this plane flying real quick!

© Copyright 2020 by CHASECHECK LTD - All rights reserved.

The content contained within this book may not be reproduced, duplicated or transmitted without direct written permission from the author or the publisher.

Under no circumstances will any blame or legal responsibility be held against the publisher, or author, for any damages, reparation, or monetary loss due to the information contained within this book. Either directly or indirectly.

Legal Notice:

This book is copyright protected. This book is only for personal use. You cannot amend, distribute, sell, use, quote or paraphrase any part, or the content within this book, without the consent of the author or publisher.

Disclaimer Notice:

Please note the information contained within this document is for educational and entertainment purposes only. All effort has been executed to present accurate, up to date, and reliable, complete information. No warranties of any kind are declared or implied. Readers acknowledge that the author is not engaging in the rendering of legal, financial, medical or professional advice. The content within this book has been derived from various sources. Please consult a licensed professional before attempting any techniques outlined in this book.By reading this document, the reader agrees that under no circumstances is the author responsible for any losses, direct or indirect, which are incurred as a result of the use of information contained within this document, including, but not limited to, — errors, omissions, or inaccuracies.

CHAPTER ONE

IT'S NOT A COINCIDENCE!

Journey to Self about Spirituality

The possession of knowledge does not kill the sense of wonder and mystery. There is always more mystery.

~Anais Nin

What's NOT a coincidence? You're probably asking, or you remember what the second paragraph of the introduction of this book says. It's nothing profound; you can check it out for yourselves.

Checked it out? Ok great. Now another question pops up. Why is it not a coincidence? It's not a coincidence that those things happen because there's something beyond what the eyes, ears, skin, nose, and tongue can see, hear, feel smell, and taste. Yup! It's beyond the five human senses.

According to Anais Nin, *"There is always more mystery."* 'Cus there is! I know that many strange things have happened in your life, and you can't just let it pass as "coincidence" or just "science?" Nah. not at all, young woman. There's gotta be something beyond what we can see which plays a massive role in the day-to-day affairs of our lives. And if we don't pay utmost attention to what it is and its demands, we will find ourselves at life's crossroads. We devote ourselves to learning about this simple concept at a loss on what to do and how to get by specific problems. It's not rocket science, and understanding it already sets you on achieving self-discovery. With self-discovery comes endless possibilities of stable physical and mental well-being.

You're probably saying, *"There's a lot to fight for. We're being discriminated against as women, and we should fight against that. What are you coming to say about some spiritual blablabla? Are we fighting ghosts?"* I'm here to tell you that the space you ought to create for your self-care, physical of course, but mostly mental, is like a shortcut to getting out of that bubble of self-pity. That's what you need to get past the demeaning remarks and all that discrimination you go through every day. You definitely won't fight them, will you? Trust me; they won't even stop if you do.

Now let's move on to the burning question. I think I've kept you waiting for quite a long time.

What is Spirituality?

The word "spirituality" has no specific definition, nor can it be defined through any rigid approach. There is no generally accepted meaning of spirituality because that same word could mean a different thing entirely when placed in another context.

I'll be repeating myself for probably the second or third time when I say that spirituality in this context is void of any form of religion or beliefs by a particular group of people. It has to do with the self. Just you in the room with no one else.

In the most straightforward words, I can find, spirituality is the search for one's inner wealth. There are so many definitions; trust me, it's not Chemistry or Math. Every author has their particular view of the subject, and with spirituality being relative, it would be out of place to say that one's definition is wrong and another right.

What Defines Your Happiness?

Many people find meaning in material stuff, millions in their bank account, and the number of followers on their Instagram page, engagements on Twitter, and many other things. If we look at such things from the world's view, they are things to be happy about. Who doesn't want a truckload of dollars in his account? But you need to ask yourself. "Should those be the only things that define my happiness?" If your answer is yes, you have to take a step back and reason what the purpose of life is.

If the number of followers you have on social media is your criteria for happiness, let me show you what your life could look like.

These followers are people you do not know personally, and no matter how you try to interact with them over social media by any means you wish, you'll never know who they are. These are not the kind of people I'd advise you to revolve your entire life around. Let me tell you why. There's a quote I came across while scrolling through TikTok some time ago, and it was from the 2002 Spiderman Movie or something like that. It read.

"But the one thing they love more than a hero is to see a hero fail, fall, die trying. They will eventually hate you despite everything you've done for them."

Those were the words of a villain in the movie, and I know we've got that cliché opinion about nothing good coming out from villains and stuff like that, but there's truth in what they say sometimes. I hope I'm not digressing, don't be carried away. Please, I've got the point to make.

We've all seen Hip Hop and Hollywood stars being "dragged" on Social Media probably because of a mistake they made or maybe not even a mistake, just some stuff that doesn't resonate well with the crowd. They receive a lot of backlashes, even death threats! Yes! That's how far people can go to prove a point forgetting that they're also humans and make mistakes.

You can imagine the emotional havoc such an occasion would wreak on the individual if they are constantly seeking validation from social media. They'd go into depression for months, and the so-called followers would not be there to comfort them.

You see! That's just how it is! It happens like that most of the time, and it's a cycle; it's not on yourself. I might have strayed a little, but it's a small price for salvation. I've made a point. It's your life, your book, and you'll not allow some uncouth fellow to write what you don't want to be written on it!

I could list things that you're not supposed to hinge your happiness on and what it'll result in when you do, but then, we're all about spirituality here, so let's keep the train moving. After reading through, you should be asking yourself now. "What defines my happiness?" Sit tight; we'll get to it.

What Should Define Your Happiness?

Are you wondering why it is all about happiness and not spirituality? Or you're just having fun moving on. If you're on either side, you're not wrong. Everything would eventually connect, and the message would become apparent.

I'll tell you why I've been all about happiness for some time.

I believe the goal of every single human on earth is to be happy.

Happiness is a common factor in the world. Everyone is running here and there, looking for cash, a lover, that degree, that job, and what have you? They're so much and can be specific too. You're looking for all those in pursuit of happiness. Well… I'd agree that most of these things are needed to live a comfortable and happy life. But what about those who have them in abundance and are still not satisfied. And you can't even ask me how I know they're not happy because you know too. We've seen bloody rich people take their own lives; if they were pleased, they wouldn't take it. I want to let you know that if you're searching for happiness in material things, you'll never find it because you're searching in the wrong place. This is not a call for you to be lazy and not go after these things if you choose to. (And when I say "go after these things," I mean legally. That should be a topic for some other time) it would help if you went for what you want, I support that, but when you neglect the things you need to pursue what you want to achieve your customized "happiness," you're going to get it all wrong.

Happiness is within. When you find your inner wealth, you've found true happiness, where spirituality comes to play.

In finding happiness, you have nothing to do with Social Media. This cannot be overemphasized.

You don't need any validation from your boss, friend, your lover, not even your religious leaders!

Strong black woman, happiness is found within, and understanding your spirituality is the only way you can do that.

I believe all dots have been connected. Or is something missing, dear?

What's the Essence of Spirituality?

As humans, we grow and evolve in the physical sense. As we grow in those areas, we need to tweak our minds and souls to be in sync. The maturing of the mind doesn't happen of its own accord as the body does. That's why we can have old yet foolish people.

As we mature, we figure out the need for certain things and the things we don't need. I'd use myself as an example here. I realized the need to be Independent when I started maturing and seeing things through my parents' eyes, who took responsibility for every aspect of my wellbeing.

Also, as I matured, I figured that I shouldn't be in any argument concerning how I live my life. I did it a lot as a child. When there was a disagreement between me and someone else concerning how certain things are done, I would argue, imposing my opinion on the other party. But then, as I grew, I realized that everyone is entitled to their opinion and choices, and setting mine on someone else was just over the edge.

It took a lot of time before I could finally adapt to this lifestyle because sometimes, even what I consider immoral would be expected of many people, and I'd be like, "Phew! You are one old-fashioned little boy, huh?" And then I'd lock my lips with my fingers and keep moving.

A lot of people get more frustrated as they mature. But that's not how it's supposed to be, and you beautiful black women are not supposed to be among that percentage of people.

Don't get me wrong, adulthood is a very crazy phase of your life that you have to be in forever, but that shouldn't make you crazy. We need a considerable level of self-consciousness to get through life as an adult, and how do you develop that? Spirituality!

Searching for that thing in your inside that gives you meaning is the best life hack you'll ever hear of.

How did it help me? I said earlier that I had to develop a resistance to arguing with people about how they should live their lives and trying to impose my style of living on them. I realized how toxic that was and how it adversely affected my state of being so much that instead of thinking about my life and what I could do to move forward and make it better, I started thinking about how wrong people were in living their lives. With these thoughts continuously ringing in my head, I became overly judgmental and always looked for a fault in everything people did around me. I was a wet blanket, carrying negative energy everywhere I went. And about people noticing I was there, they quickly left or avoided speaking with me. For some time, I thought that I was still right and whatever they did was wrong, and I didn't care. Not until the people I loved started avoiding me did I realize that I was supposed to draw the line and stop playing God. I was beginning to allow that toxic trait to destroy me and my relationship with the people I loved. I had to go back to the drawing board to search deep within. I asked myself many questions (we'll be looking at that later on), put myself in the shoes of the others, and realized that something was off.

I got it all fixed up, and everything changed. I began to judge less. Hence I worried less. It started from within. I felt this freedom of mind was second to none, and it gave me a new outlook on life. Even when someone else was starting the argument, I'd say, "OK. You already won before the fight started. Congratulations" I still do this, and it works perfectly for me. You need to experience the peace that comes with fixing a spiritual problem in your life. (This is not an exorcism, please.)

I've probably said too much, and you're starting to feel I haven't responded to the question in the sub-heading. I have, but I'd give you something much more straightforward, something you can take.

The essence of spirituality is to help you seek a meaningful connection with something beyond the physical, which causes positive emotions such as peace, contentment, gratitude, and acceptance. These emotions help you battle negative emotions such as pride, greed, hate, etc. Spirituality can be seen as a means to an end; there's no limit to what the black woman can achieve when embracing her spirituality.

Who Is A Spiritual Person?

You probably have a picture of Bishop draped in a white cassock with a collar at the neck, holding a giant bible in his right hand and a cross-shaped staff in his left hand. Or an Imam with full beards and a perfectly tied turban around his head, with an equally long flowing garment. But then ask yourself this question. Don't you think it rather strange to define who a spiritual person is by their physical appearance? I mean, take a look at the antithesis! The opposite of the word "spiritual" is "physical." And then someone defines who a spiritual person is by physical features? That's just absurd! One of the craziest perceptions in life that has been unfortunately normalized if you ask me.

But then, who indeed is a spiritual person? It's simple.

A spiritual person has a love for herself and others as a priority. In this context, that's all it takes to be a spiritual person. You can be clad in the purest of whites, holding the enormous bibles, and still not being spiritual. In the same vein, you can be dressed like a gangster with tattoos all over your skin and piercings and still be a spiritual person. (Please note that this is not a piece of fashion advice.)

Are we together, my lady?

Spirituality is mainly lived as a personal and internal experience. There are no rules, unlike many other religions. No one has the right to punish you for mistakes made because the whole process is internalized. Rather than punish yourself for your mistakes, you consider those mistakes fundamental for growth and progress. Yeah, you turn that vinegar into wine and keep on moving!

When a black woman embraces her spirituality, she doesn't need to mull over the past and condemn herself for her bad choices; she lives in the present and implements the lessons learned.

We will be looking at one more issue before I draw the curtains close for this chapter.

Spirituality and Emotional Health

As you go through this book, you'd notice that most of the recommendations on cultivating spirituality are similar to those recommended for improving emotional fitness and well-being. This is because spirituality and emotional health are intertwined and influence each other.

You may be asking what the relationship between Spirituality and Emotional Health is. It's simple math.

As I said earlier in this book, spirituality seeks a meaningful connection with something beyond the physical. Yes.

On the other hand, emotional health is about cultivating the right frame of mind, which can widen one's vision to recognize and connect with something beyond the physical.

The underlying relationship between spirituality and emotional health is that improved emotional health will open one's eyes to spirituality. I'll explain briefly.

When you've progressed to a certain level in improving your emotional health, you begin to see the need to connect to something greater. It sounds a little bit absurd in theory, but practically, it's not out of the norm. We could also say that spirituality is seeking advancement in the stability of our emotional health.

In the next chapter, my main focus will be on understanding yourself and understanding spirituality for yourself. What's all the knowledge when you can't use it to improve yourself? Such knowledge, I'd consider, a waste.

I know we're still together, stay with me on this one and let's help ourselves improve the quality of the lives of our black women.

Key Points

- Spirituality is not all about religion
- Nothing is a coincidence
- The search for inner wealth is the only way to genuine happiness

- Social media should never define what happiness is to you.
- Embracing your spirituality is the most significant life hack there is.
- Physical qualities do not discern spirituality.
- Finding and embracing one's spirituality is an internalized process.
- Mistakes from your past are lessons in disguise. Learn.
- Spirituality and emotional health are distinct but connected.
- Embrace your spirituality, black woman!

CHAPTER TWO

KNOW YOURSELF!

Understanding Spirituality for Yourself.

"Your pain is the breaking of the shell that encloses your understanding."

– Kahlil Gibran

Now it's great that we know what spirituality is all about, the essence, and its relationship with other aspects of our lives, such as our emotional health. But you see, spirituality can't mean the same thing to everybody, and if you don't know and understand yourself, you're probably putting all of your energy in the wrong place. It's of utmost importance that you do not use any other person's spirituality as a standard while searching for your inner wealth.

Wait a sec... is that even possible? Not in my book because spirituality is an internalized process. You can't even peep into the reality of someone else's spirituality. If you think you do, then you're looking at something else.

People only show you what they want you to see.

Spirituality starts from the inside and then starts to manifest outwardly. But then, a lot of people know how to fake smiles! Have you ever come across a fruit that looks all yellow and attractive on the outside, and when you mistake biting into it, your tongue suffers the sour taste? That's how a lot of people live their lives. Alive on the outside but slowly dying on the inside, so if you're looking at someone from afar, living the good life, smiling and you know, all the stuff people do to hide their problems, you'd think that, oh yeah, that man's got it all worked out spiritually, physically and the sort. While you may be a hundred percent right, you may also be blindly wrong! People go through a lot and go through more to hide their pain. Not the point we're driving at, just an illustration to show that you can't possibly mimic one's spirituality because it most definitely won't fit.

The only solution is knowing, finding, and understanding your spiritual version.

So what do we do to know? The first thing you need to do is look up on Google, search for your Zodiac sign, and bingo! You got it all fixed up. Easy as pie, right? If it were that simple, I'd not bother fighting my sleep to get this across. How would you explain that they'd have the same attitude and mindset because people were born on the same day? Even twins would think differently from each other! I've come across many of them, and none of them I've seen share the same attributes or way of life. That means the Zodiac signs would not be the most accurate tool to determine such aspects of human life. It's way beyond that, sister.

What if you start by asking yourself specific questions?

In the journey to self-discovery, asking questions is vital, and when I mean asking questions, I do not mean asking other people questions. I suggest asking ourselves to ascertain what sort of people we indeed are, and as long as we're not doing anything wrong to anybody, we ought to embrace who we are and work on our flaws. Not a one-day process, but it is worth it in the end.

So what are some of these questions we need to ask ourselves?

Ever asked yourself. *"Am I a good person?"*

This kind of question is what people would ask other people and expect to hear sweet stuff like, *"Yeah, you're the sweetest person I know,"* *"You're so humble,"* *"Such a great smiler,"* and you know, your head begins to swell for few minutes, but when you leave the area, they start talking shit about you.

Let me reiterate this, ladies. In discovering and understanding yourself, don't you ever give any duty to another person, not even your clergy or religious leaders? The process is all you and no one else. Give it to someone else, and all you will have are errors and misconceptions about yourself. Wild, isn't it?

So what do you do?

You sit down, black lady—just you, in your private space. Make sure you're comfortable and not in a funny shape. I'm not joking. I mean serious business, you hear me?

And then throw the question to yourself. *"Elena, Kate, Grace, Sophia. Are you a good person?"* If you can do that now, do it and notice how you'll feel. After asking yourself the question, you begin to flood your mind with so many events, and then you start to reflect on so many choices you've made, so many actions you've taken, and how those choices and actions affected and are affecting you in the long run. What do you feel about those choices?

Was it something you gave, or something you refused to provide, an encouraging comment you made, or a depressing one? Put yourself in the shoes of people you relate with day after day and try to find out how you'll react to certain things you've done. You're going to come out with answers at the end of the process. And the answer will mostly not be a yes or no answer, and this is what it will look like.

You'll figure out that we have casually done excellent and evil in the process of living. So the answer can't come out as a Yes or No answer. Let's not lie to ourselves; it won't, black ladies.

What will be the result is the need for improvement. Yes! Self-improvement. You'll find out that, ok Uhm… I said that I wasn't supposed to speak to the young guy at the market, and I needed to make sure I didn't say that to someone else because if it were said to me, I'd feel distraught. And then you'll probably put that down in your diary or something and hop on to the next. It's an everyday process. You can't possibly finish questioning yourself for a day. It's continuous. It goes on and on and on till we finally leave the earth.

Concerning what our topic is in this chapter, as you keep on questioning yourself and working on setting things right, a constant will appear. What do I mean? Probably before now, everybody has an opinion of you except you. Whether they're wrong or right, they do.

But then you probably don't because you haven't scrutinized yourself and tried to act along a line of refinement. So when you eventually do, for week 1, week 2, and week 3, you'll begin to see a pattern that gets better as time goes by. Then you can precisely pinpoint what kind of a person you are or aren't—good, bad, or most definitely something else peculiar to you and only.

Embracing our spirituality ought to lead to self-improvement, and this is what questioning yourself can do. When you take this as an everyday practice, you begin to connect with your spiritual side. There's good in everyone. Inner riches! Find it, act on it and live a stress-free life. At first, trying to keep up with it every day will be tasking, but I tell you that it will be worth it as each day goes by. Trust me.

What other question can you ask yourself in your journey to knowing and understanding spirituality for yourself?

You can ask yourself. *"Do things happen for a reason?"*

Well... hell yes, they do! Everything happens for a reason. You can't develop a specific sense of why something terrible happened to you, but there's a general notion of why things happen the way they do.

And that's to make you learn. There's no manual to life, woman. You live and learn, and you know as you live. So whatever stuff happens to you that got you messed up, it's for you to learn. And whatever good stuff that happened to you is for you to know as well.

When you ask yourself such a question, and you answer it yourself, you begin to have a different outlook on life.

You can pick out some events that happened due to a mistake you made that took its toll on you, and after asking yourself if it happened for a reason which it did, other questions begin to pop in. That's how it works. You begin to ask yourself again.

"What did I learn from this event?

Have I made the same mistake since?

How has it affected my life?

Am I a better person now than before?"

Do you see how it connects? Oh well! I think asking yourself questions is one underrated activity, don't you think so? Look at how I've managed to x-ray my life by just asking myself simple questions and getting the best possible answer I can get from myself. Never forget, it's only you in the room and anyone else.

Please tell me how you wouldn't understand a topic at school, let's say Uhm… Negligence in law. Then every day, you make a note to ask questions on it.

What is Negligence? What constitutes negligence, and so on? It's impossible not to understand it better than you will when you sit there.

It applies to our lives, women. Ask yourself questions and understand yourself more because that's the cheat code.

I hope you're hanging in there, my black queen?

Let's look at another question we can ask ourselves. This is going to be the last one.

This question is more like a concluding question after you've gone to great lengths to understand who you are.

Ask yourself.

"How can I live my life in the best possible way?"

I don't think there'll be much to talk about here. Be the you that you understand. You'll be out of shape sometimes. And you're going to be like…

"Damn, I don't understand what I'm doing here!"

Sometimes it's not out of the norm to feel out of place. But it's unhealthy to feel that way for too long. You're going to improve with time. And remember that you compete with yourself and no one else.

That's how to live your life in the best possible way. Come out a better version of yourself every day. Your down days will only make you come out better when it's over.

Never stop being You!

Carl Jung said, *"The privilege of a lifetime is to become who you really are."*

Those words struck me when I came across them at a particular time in my life when I wasn't exactly who I was supposed to be, and I knew it. When you're not who you are, no one else will notice more than you will. If you're reading this book right now and you're not who you are, this paragraph should strike hard because you know that you're not living the life you ought to live. And every night, you sit down and ask why you've been so empty and unfulfilled in your pursuit of happiness. Do you know what's interesting?

You could be in a mansion, on vacation at a private beach, on a private ship, or on a private plane; you can be living what people would say is your best life and still be perturbed about a missing piece that you're yet to find.

Embrace your spirituality and give yourself that privilege that Carl Jung spoke of. You've worked way too hard not to be living the life that frees your mind, soul, and body.

Mistakes

Mistakes play a massive role in helping you understand yourself more. Especially the ones that happen in your mind. One that no one has access to. I'll give an example. Maybe you have a misconception about someone because of what you saw them do or what someone told you, and then cultivate some hate against someone who probably doesn't know you. Except you're a robot, you'd feel terrible if you find out that the one you hate hasn't done anything wrong or doesn't even have anything against you and probably loves you.

Allow me to give another example. It's just like a man who marries a woman who fails to provide him with a child, and then he goes for other women making it two or three wives who now bear him children, fortunately for him. Then he begins to despise his first wife because she has been labeled "barren." He says harsh words to her and could even go physical with her. Although in this case, it wouldn't be an entirely internal mistake, and people who are close enough would notice.

Nevertheless, it doesn't change that it all starts with the mind, making it an internal mistake. If life decides to happen and such a man falls sick or loses all his money, properties, and other assets and valuables.

The only person who remains to take care of him is the first wife, whom he despises because she bore him no child. That man would undoubtedly wish the earth would open up and swallow him. Don't you think so?

And if it so happens that he recovers from the setback, he's undoubtedly going to learn a lesson, wouldn't he? Yes, he would! Such a person would ask himself various questions (remember, right?) And when he finds answers to those questions, he would've unlocked a side to himself that he had never known or had access to. And when he does, if he's genuinely remorseful for what he did, self-improvement kicks in. The man will never want to feel as horrible as he did when he figured out he made the big mistake and would try as much as possible to make sure such a thing doesn't repeat itself.

Learn! Don't Linger!

The peace that comes with knowing and understanding yourself can't even be imagined. I tell you the truth. When you know yourself, even the mistakes you make that cost you a lot become a stepping stone to learning something new about life.

You know, when people have made mistakes and have failed in life, the problem isn't about whether they've discovered the lesson to be learned or not. Also, the problem isn't about whether they've learned the study from the mistakes or not because certainly when a similar situation like that presents happens in the future. They would've been wise enough to say, *"Ok, I did it this way the last time, and it landed me in some unfortunate circumstances, so I'll do it this way instead."*

But then the issue is that you're hanging your head over for too long! I wish I could emphasize that enough. Too long, queen! And why the hell is that? You never thought you could make such a mistake? 'Course we're humans. We make mistakes.

Ridiculous ones sometimes, to be frank. It's in our nature to do so. We've seen prominent figures do so too. So why should you be hard on yourself because of a silly mistake? No offense, but that's just silly all the more. You're probably enjoying the sympathy from those who love and care and want to see you back on your feet soon as possible? Why not show them that you're worth loving, and of what use is the love of other people when you're busy hating yourself? Get back up and smile on the faces of those who love you.

Let Go! Please don't force it!

Winding up this chapter, I'd love to refer to the words of Ramana Maharshi where he said,

"Let what comes come. Let what goes go. Find out what remains."

As we progress, we acquire, and we shed. What makes us who we are is remaining when the trimming is done.

I believe that sometimes, we look back into our past lives and remember some things we had which we have no more, and then we probably fake a short smile or something. It can be a person or an interest.

Make sure you don't force any of them. Telling yourself the truth will also help a lot with that.

Life is full of surprises, my beautiful woman. We may think that something's going to stay forever and then it eventually doesn't. And we may also feel like, *"No, I don't need this."* And that's what finally stays. Learn to be flexible. Flexibility is undoubtedly one of the most challenging steps to knowing ourselves because of the issue of attachment. Of course, it hurts losing a loved one, but then you'll get used to living without that person, and life goes on. Sadly though.

What about your interests? Maybe you find out something you're interested in, could be a skill or something else. A time comes when you're no longer feeling the vibe, and you're not interested anymore.
It's not because you're lazy. It just doesn't fit, and we're so lucky to have been blessed with such complex bodies that we know when we're no longer cut out for this stuff, and we'd have to severe the times and the connection and the connection we already have with such a thing.

You'll lose a lot of things eventually, but you're not going to lose everything. Focus on those things that remain. They are a part of what makes you "the you" of your dreams.

Key Points

- Spirituality cannot be the same for everybody
- People only show you what they want you to see.
- Constantly question yourself
- Everything happens for a reason
- Never give the duty of ascertaining your spirituality to someone else.
- Understand that there are going to be a lot of setbacks.
- Be yourself anyway.
- Never get used to staying on the ground
- Don't force things
- Focus on the things that remain.

CHAPTER THREE

IT'S ALL IN YOUR HANDS

"It is not in the stars to hold our destiny but in ourselves."

– William Shakespeare

As a kid, I used to look at the stars and pray to them for wealth, fame, and all other "good things of life." If you've got kids that still do that, please allow them to because being a kid is what we all wish for now as adults, and you wouldn't want to interfere with that phase of their lives because when it goes, it's gone forever.

However, you'd have to make sure you let them know at the right time that the stars hold no destiny of theirs. You've got to make them look at their hands and say to them. "Look… you see those two hands; those are what holds your destiny, not the stars." Although they might get a hint before you tell them, they probably won't believe that they've got so much to do, I mean… *"why do I have to do so much when I've got my mama?"* Haha! Funny, isn't it. Funny, hard truth.

Your kids aren't the main focus, though; I just thought I should chip in some parental advice and lighten the mood. After reading this, you owe your kids a duty to let them know this at the right time. If this is not the right time for them, then take a chill pill and focus on yourself. At least for now.

So, where did we stop?

Your destiny, your future. You hold it in your hands, and this knowledge makes you realize that you've got no one but yourself and that your well-being should come first. Not disputing that you should also care for those you love because loving yourself is the first step to loving others. You can't give what you don't have, can you?

For some people, the realization creeps up on them, little by little, day by day, slowly until it's full-blown, and you can't run away from it anymore. But for some other people like me, it came banging on my door, didn't even wait for me to open it before it broke the door, came straight to me, and hijacked me. I almost had a heart attack when it suddenly dawned on me that I would be the one responsible for my well-being in the long run.

I can still remember how it happened. I was in high school, looking for some money for a project, and then I went to my father to ask him for the money.

I went to him and was like,

"Uhm... Dad, I need some money for a school project." Then he replied

"How much will it cost me?"

"Just ten bucks, Dad." Then he raised his head to look at me.

"Just ten bucks, huh? Alright. So what's going to happen if I don't give you ten bucks for your project?"

I was confused. What's this man talking about? Did I need to go through all these for just ten bucks? It was unlike my Dad. Then I replied, trying to be sarcastic because I thought he was only joking

"Well... if you don't give me the ten bucks, I can't finish the school project, and then I'll fail the course." My father flashed a half-smile at me and got up from where he sat and asked me.

"And how much will that cost me?"

The room went silent, and the only sound I could hear was my father's feet walking out of the room while I stood there thinking about how much my father hated me. Haha

Later that night, he called me to the same room and had me sit down to listen to him.

He told me that he had a responsibility to take care of me and whether I was going to fail or not mattered less to him because, over the years, he had narrowed his purpose to taking care of his family, and nothing would change that.

My father wasn't the one to wait for his kids to grow before him "reaped the fruits of his labor," all he cared about was carrying out his responsibilities till he died.

He said to me

"Look here, child; If you fall, I'm not the one who gets a scar. It's you who does."

After that, he handed the ten bucks to me and went to bed.

It was like I was struck by lightning. I couldn't sleep that night. I stayed awake all through thinking about how life would be without my father to give me ten bucks for a school project, and since that night, I was all in for anything that would improve my life in all aspects. I realized that nobody would be responsible for my success or failure, but for me, so I had to make it work for myself.

I want every black woman also to realize this. Her destiny is in her hands, so she should work towards her progress, no matter how small, reminding her of the need to connect with her spiritual self. Being a success is not just by wealth and fame. A father who has it all should be more worried about his child than a father who doesn't. Why am I saying this? Most rich people care about ensuring that their families eat well, are well clothed, and have the "best things in life."

(You should know why I put things like this in a quote.) But then they neglect the things that matter the most. What about the spiritual and mental well-being of the child?

They know that one day, the child will be independent, and even if you give a child the whole world without letting her know that she needs to be connected and acquainted with her spiritual self, it will yield more when you donate to charity instead. A spiritually unsound person will be an unsafe person in the physical realm, and then money might not be able to help such a person.

Instead, it'll destroy them more. Or don't you know that

putting the right thing in the wrong hands makes the right thing bad and causes more harm than good? I guess you do now.

So when you know that you owe a duty to yourself and your child or children to make sure they have the things that matter, let the drive to learn more about your inner wealth increase. After reading this book, pick up another one, reflect, practice, manifest, and you will see progress. And when you see improvement, don't stop there and let it get into your head. Make more progress. It's only unfair to yourself when you're working hard to get something done and stop when you get to the middle. Why did you stop? How does stopping benefit you?

I watched Steve Harvey on TikTok the other day, and he was saying, *"If you're going through hell, keep going because why would you want to stop in hell?"*

Or why would you want to turn back, only to go through the same hell again later on because no matter how hard you try, you can only run away from your problems when you're no longer breathing. If you can remember, I wrote in the previous chapter that one should ask him or herself whether things happen for a reason. You must know that you're passing through hell for a reason, and the only way you can understand why is to walk through till the end. Humans want answers to many questions, and they forget that most answers lie in what they're running away from. Some questions can't be answered by anyone else except you.

Take that problem you're going through as a question and work the solution from start to finish. And see how fulfilled you'll be when you finally arrive at the answer. It's so much fun when we live our lives like that. Don't you want to have stories to tell? Imagine how satisfied you'll be when you tell your children how you pulled through that challenging situation you thought you would die in. You'll become a superhero spreading hope

People may have answers to many questions you have to ask, but for some, only you know their answers, and you have to answer them to move forward in life.

LIVING ISN'T EASY

I want to use this medium to thank all black ladies worldwide. Wherever you are right now, know that you're highly appreciated by some random guy who badly wants to see you overcome depression and embrace who you are and some guy who wants to see you win.

Maybe I've been kind of hard on you in some parts of this book, though I try my best not to; this is to tell you that I understand the pain you're going through. We're in a world where women are hated for being robust, bold, and beautiful. All of which tell the story of a black woman.

Even a thirteen-year-old knows that life isn't easy. So this is not me about to tell you what you don't already know. I'm more ignorant than I think you are if I think I am. But this is me trying to tell you to embrace what you know would make life more bearable for you.

Now you can't physically fight those trying to make your life miserable. They're going to lock you up and make your life even more tragic, but then you have a defense—a very competent and reliable one.

Shut your eyes and ears to the toxic crowd; otherwise, you'll be distracted. Remind yourself that you're your only hope, and if you can't do something to help yourself, nothing anyone else does to help will suffice. The anxiety is just an illusion. Walk past it like a mirage by constantly looking at the brighter side. You're permitted to sulk, but not for long. There's no time to do that; you've got lives to touch and souls to heal. You can't mend others when you're broken; you'll only break them the more. Heal yourself and then be healing to others. Isn't that a part of what spirituality is about? Spreading love and light? It most definitely is.

So you've got to know yourself, woman. This chapter is like an extension of the previous one because when you realize that your destiny is in your hands, you'll have to make sure you tick the essential boxes to get you through life. One of which is knowing yourself and understanding spirituality for yourself, and not letting anybody fill you with fallacies. When you do that, you improve yourself and everyone around you, and you're fulfilled, just like I am for writing this book.

Never forget, in this race, it is you before anyone else. Knowing that women would most likely put someone else before themselves, this cannot, therefore, be overemphasized.

Key Points

- It's all in your hands.

- You can't give out what you don't have.
- Take every step to progress, no matter how small.
- Wealth and fame are not all there is to success and fulfillment.
- Putting the right thing in the wrong hands makes the right thing bad and causes more harm than good.
- It doesn't make any sense to stop while walking through hell.
- If you can't do something to help yourself, nothing anyone else does to help will suffice.
- You're permitted to sulk, but not for long.
- Walk past anxiety by looking at the brighter side.
- You can't mend others when you're broken.
- Spread love and light!

CHAPTER FOUR

BUILDING UP YOUR SPIRITUAL ENERGY

"Believe in your infinite potential. Your only limitations are those you set upon yourself."

– Roy T. Bennett

Ever tried working out? Some of you should have. I wish I could make a graphical representation of how stuff like that usually goes. I can't, but one thing is sure, and you must know that it's not a one-way journey.

You start the first day feeling pumped, excited, and ready to get that body in shape. What is it you don't do? Push-ups, pull-ups, lifting weights, what else? You do everything on the first day, and if you're lucky enough, the vibe follows you on to the next day and the next. You probably keep it up for a week, and as the following week approaches, you feel the vibe beginning to dwindle. Why? You're in severe pain, tired of the diet, or busy and have other things to pursue, or laziness has hit you already. Then you stop.

Stop? I think that's where we're going to have minor fracas here.

That's how it is; that's how it always goes. These stages must come, and then it's left for you to succumb to the pressure or be very intentional about what you want to achieve. The fact that you succumb doesn't make you less of a human, no-no-no. That's how humans are built. We got some, lost some, and then learned all we could. We want but can't have it all. Completely fine.

But then, you want to do this stuff! You want to see results! You're intentionally getting your body in shape to accentuate the magical black beauty and aesthetics already built in a black woman like you.

So despite the pain and the inconvenience, you still got that picture of the lady you want to see yourself become physically, and you don't stop. You never stop. Even when you've gotten to the point you thought you needed to, if you stop right there, you'll only be drawn back to where you started from.

I don't think it'll be out of place to relate physical workouts with building spiritual strength. Even while they're total opposites, they have similarities. You start a physical workout routine to improve your physical health while working on your spirituality guarantees an improvement in your mental health. Another similarity is that you never stop. I've said this earlier; it keeps going on and on because you start to depreciate when you stop.

As we course through this chapter, I'm going to be making a lot of references to physical workout routines since it's something almost everyone can relate to. It'll make the ride more fun and fulfilling.

Be Intentional

Two powerful words up there. You know, one doesn't need a lot of sophisticated grammar to prove a point. Any comment is powerful and holds a powerful message.

Intentionality is one virtue that everyone needs when they embark on a significant journey to self-improvement. That's one of the things that keep you on track. The picture of that desired goal you have in your head, that you look at when you wake up every morning and before you go to bed at night.

You're not doing what you do because other people do it. But because you've found out that it's something that you need to do. Before you can be intentional about something, you must have found a need for it. If not, you're just wasting your time because when it becomes hard to catch up, since you didn't find any need in it, you become lost, and you don't see any need to continue. Boom! Time and probably money wasted and nothing achieved. That's a bad investment in my books. Why not start something you can finish?

In this case, this is something we all need as humans. I spent a lot of time discussing the need to embrace our spirituality which I hope now has a firm ground in your hearts. What's next after the first step at embracing your spirituality? Don't you think there's room for growth and improvement? Of course! Nudge yourself when you're in one spot because you're not supposed to be there for long.

Being intentional will help you when you find out that you've been in one spot for quite a while. Why? You begin to realize that you're now accepting life as it comes, and you're not leading your life. Now let me tell you something. Nobody ever achieved what they wanted to achieve by accident, so you've got to be intentional while you're after building that spiritual energy.

Now I can't possibly tell you how to be intentional. You're not intentional because you're doing certain things; instead, you do certain things when you're intended. So being intentional is like a moving vehicle that drives you to go the extra mile to achieve what you want to.

Face your Challenges – Don't Whine for Long.

What doesn't kill you makes you stronger. I bet everyone is familiar with the above statement already as part of the lyrics of a song I know, and it's true. We will complain so much about how unfair life is in our life's journey. We're going to be tested many times, and when we get out of the booby-traps, we're not going to be the same person we were when we first got in there.

In the same vein, in our journey to spiritual enlightenment and fulfillment, we will face many obstacles. We will lose friends, friends who can't accept that you're gradually changing as you embrace your spirituality. You're going to have to stop doing a lot of things that would be a hindrance to your growth. A lot of things will happen that will make you question if you should even be on that path. But trust me. It only gets better. Now note that I didn't say it only gets more accessible, but better. I say this because your challenges become more challenging, and you become better. I don't know if I can call it an inverse relationship; just letting you know that you deserve all the credit for the challenges you pass through. They don't usually become more manageable; you only get better.

Now, it's ok to be scared. Am I scared of what? Afraid of the fact that challenges are going to get more complicated. When I look back at the challenges I've faced and how I overcame them, I get scared because I know that something way worse will come after, and I begin to wonder if I'm ever going to make it alive. The funny part is when I go through those challenges; It doesn't even occur to me that I thought I'd never go through them.

So yeah. Expect challenges, failures, setbacks, and trauma. But whine for a long time because there's no time. Focus your energy on getting out of it and see how strong you become.

Seek Knowledge

All the time. Never think that you can stop learning because you can't. If you try not to learn, then you know the hard way. Well, learning is learning afterward, so there you have it.

Learn from experiences. Both the ones that are yours and those that aren't, read books on spirituality like this one. Listen to people who have something to offer on the subject and watch spirituality shows. You can't get all the knowledge in one place, not that you're going to get them all at first, but at least you died trying.

Having a lot of things to do can get one messed up sometimes. So, to cushion the effect of having so much to do with little time, make a table placing priorities first and be disciplined. If you feel that you have to be on TikTok every day, make time for it and make sure what you're taking in doesn't hinder your growth as a spiritual person. A day can't contain all that you need to do? Spread it throughout your week and repeat the things on top of the list every day. The less important ones? Maybe two to three times a week. Work on your discipline with that. You're strong when you're disciplined, and you'll achieve a lot.

Evaluation

It does more good than harm to stop and reflect. You might not notice many things when you're out there making things happen. So once in a while, get in your room, lock the door, sit and meditate. Reflect. What has changed? How have I been feeling these days? How do people around me react to the change I've undergone? The answers you get are also motivating factors to keep you going. If you feel better than you were before, you will want to make it stay that way all your life.

People might have walked out of your life during the phase, but you might not be aware of it unless you reflect. Then you'll realize that.

"Oh! I don't think Matilda talks to me as she does anymore. Hmm, sad." And then you go on to see the ones that have stayed regardless, and you'll be like.

"Alright! These got my back."

Then you'll know how to treat them accordingly. It would be best if you weren't giving so much energy to those who have become uncomfortable with your change process because such people would try to talk you out of it. So please give them the space they deserve and embrace those who have found you still worthy of being in their life regardless.

How does this help build your strength? I'll tell you.

When you work with the knowledge you have gotten from self-evaluation, it builds up your spiritual strength.

I'm going to show this with an example.

When you distance yourself from the people who don't want to accept your change and embrace those who do? You'll be surrounded mainly by the people who care. And what's a better option than being surrounded by the energy you need to forge ahead in life? I'll be dwelling on this later in this book when I talk about purging yourself of evil power and people. I just wanted to emphasize the need to reflect and evaluate your growth.

Still on Evaluation...

Evaluate your thoughts about the people around you. How do you see the people around you? What do you think about them? Are you judging them? What do you feel when something good or bad happens to them? Are you bitter when they're happy? Are you glad when they're going through hell? Make sure you're not lying to yourself when you ask yourself these questions. That's also one thing that can help build up your spiritual strength. Be completely honest with yourself. It's not a hard thing to do. We actually can't even lie to ourselves. Most people shy away from the truth they've already told themselves when they know the absolute truth. So this is me urging you to be a different black woman. Tell yourself the truth because you're the only one who can.

When you've answered the questions about how you feel about people around you, ask yourself again how they would think if they could read your mind. How would you feel if you knew that a close friend had been judgmental? You'd certainly feel bad. So you know what to do. Work on that!

Many people go through a lot, and if they know that someone out there like you are rooting solidly for them, it would make them a lot better and give them reasons not to give up.

Connect with Nature

I don't think I've said anything about the relationship between spirituality and nature. When you often connect yourself with nature and Earth, you become aligned with the natural living energy. You can achieve this by spending some time outside closed doors, like eating out or even taking a stroll to see the sunrise or sunset.

The feeling you get is unexplainable, by the way, but it's worth a try. Enjoy the mild sunshine at dusk, feel the energy in the wind blow through you and appreciate nature. Some form of fulfillment comes from there. Trust me.

Acts of Service

Don't you feel good when you engage in acts of service towards your community and those around you? Let's not even take it too far. How do you feel when your friends or a relative come over to your house, and you make them feel comfortable, make them lunch or dinner, and so on? If you're not expecting anything in return, that feeling of satisfaction is priceless! One might feel burdened because they're expecting some payback. That's wrong. If you're expecting something in return for an act of service, you'll only get angry when you don't get it, which will defy the whole purpose of the action.

Keep serving. Mother Earth knows how to bless you for those acts of service.

Share the Process

Find someone who will need what you have to offer and share your journey with them. It could be your son, daughter, even a kid in the class you teach, your neighbor's child, or even grown-ups like you! Spend time telling them what you have achieved due to the bold step of embracing your spirituality. You will be shocked at many things you will learn from opening up.

On the other hand, hook up with people you know who have achieved what you're seeking to achieve. There's a lot of knowledge packed in there too. Never let anyone tell you otherwise. Knowledge is still power and will always be.

You Always Have a Choice

Don't you ever think that you do not have a choice? You always have an option to do what suits you. Exercise that power of choice every day! Don't let it control your choice no matter what happens to you. You can choose joy over sadness and depression. Whatever that guy had done to you, always remember that you've got a choice to choose forgiveness over revenge. You can choose love over hate.

It's your choice not in certain situations, but always exercise your power of choice in all conditions.

Exercising the power of choice gives one an edge over their emotions and saves them from a lot of trouble caused by making decisions in the heat of a moment.

Count your Blessings

Don't be so overwhelmed by life's problems that you forget to identify the blessings it has brought your way. It'll be unfair to focus more on the bad than the good. If you're going to dwell on things that caused you so much pain and agony, why not on things that brought a smile to even it out? You'll only be damaged at the end of the day if you count your setbacks.

Victor M. Parachin, in an article he wrote, **"21 Ways to Build a Stronger Spiritual Life,"** suggested a "count-your-blessing" exercise to try for a week.

According to him;

At the end of the first day, identify a blessing that came to you from a family member. At the end of the second day, a blessing from a neighbor. On the third day, from a friend. On the fourth day, from a work colleague. On the fifth day, from a stranger. Sixth day, from a child. On the seventh day, a blessing came from an "enemy."

Check that out and notice the changes within a month.

Be Reliable

It would help if you were someone you could count on. Have you made a to-do list for tomorrow? Make sure you attempt to do up to Fifty percent of what you planned, if not a hundred. Remember I told you that it starts from within. People can rely on you as time passes if you can rely on yourself!

It's all for self-improvement, and it starts to manifest in due time.

Be Grateful

Never forget to be grateful for growth. Look back on those things that have happened in your life, the good, the bad, and the ugly. And be thankful for how they've helped shape you to become who you presently are. You may not be where you want to be. Do we even get to where we want to be in life? That could be relative, but I don't think so. So you've got to be grateful you're not where you used to be. That's like a form of encouragement that one day, you're still going to look back on today and be like;

"Phew! I made it past there then, and now I'm here, hoping to make it past somewhere else in the future."

That defines growth, woman! And don't you ever forget to be grateful for it.

To conclude this chapter, I'm going to remind you that you're only human, and you should not be discouraged by your inability to carry out most of all the stuff I've talked about here.

Show up every day, and you'll see that it indeed gets better with time.

Keep your eyes on the goal and when you're struggling to meet it, remember that if not for anything at all, you have or you're going to have kids that will need the knowledge and experience you've garnered by deciding to venture into taking your spirituality seriously.

They don't have to suffer what you suffered and what's more fulfilling than knowing that you've got them covered even as a mother?

You're superhuman, knowing that you've got something to offer more than the average!

KEY POINTS

- The journey always starts easy and gets challenging as you progress.

- Nobody ever achieved what they wanted to accomplish by accident. They did so because they were intentional.

- Always remember, what doesn't kill you makes you stronger. It doesn't get easier; you become stronger.

- Expect challenges, failures, setbacks, and trauma. Prepare to move on as soon as possible as well.

- Don't ever think you can stop learning. It never ends.

- Always look back, see how far you've come, and note the changes. In essence, evaluate yourself.

- Any opportunity you get to serve humanity, don't take it for granted. Serve

- Share your experiences with people who need to learn from you and people you can learn from.

- Never forget you wield the power of your choice.

- Always be grateful for progress.

CHAPTER FIVE

LIVING YOUR SPIRITUALITY

"Happiness cannot be traveled to, owned, earned, worn, or consumed. Happiness is the spiritual experience of living every minute with love, grace, and gratitude."

– Denis Waitley

Living your spirituality is associated with what was discussed in the previous chapter, building one's spiritual strength. These two things go hand in hand. Every concern under spirituality is closely linked together, whether inversely or directly. While trying to live our spirituality, we're also building up our spiritual strength, so this relationship is direct.

Now, what do we mean by living our spirituality?

I want to refer you back to when we said that the essence of spirituality is to help you seek a meaningful connection with something beyond the physical, which causes positive emotions such as peace, contentment, gratitude, and acceptance. These emotions help you battle negative emotions such as pride, greed, hate, etc.

Now, look at where I'm headed. As much as embracing your spirituality is more of an internal activity than an external one, what's going to be the proof that you've improved yourself? You can't tell people you've embraced your spirituality when your actions contradict what you preach. No one's going to take you seriously. You've not even taken yourself seriously in the first place because you've not incorporated what you have learned into your everyday life. That's quite unfortunate if you ask me.

So how then do you live your spirituality? Hang on, and I'll walk you through some ways you can live your spirituality to the fullest.

Acknowledge the Unknown

One truth remains. There's a lot more to life than we see every day. And no matter how "realistic" we try to be every day, there's something that happens to us that we cannot explain. That we don't see it does not mean it does not exist. Even if we don't see it, we've got to acknowledge that it's there and responsible for many things that happen to us. We would never know what it is, that's why it's called the unknown, but when we live our lives having in mind that something beyond our understanding exists, there'll be no need to get worked up so much about life. That's one benefit of embracing your spirituality. Your worry reduces, and peace takes over.

Forgive Yourself

In the earlier chapters of this book, I told you that we shouldn't let our setbacks hold us longer than they should. What's the first step to letting go? Forgiving yourself. We're all humans, and we make mistakes.

No matter how grave the error was (except you've willingly taken a life, entirely over the edge to me.) No one has the right to take your life. You don't even have the right to bring your own life. So what do you do? Go about living with self-inflicted pain and emotional trauma? I say no! I don't see a black woman doing that, and it's not going to start with you. Remember that you're dealing with yourself here, so you're allowed to make mistakes, and you should forgive yourself completely for them so you can move forward.

Forgive Others

Since we're trying to live our spirituality now, it's not about us anymore. Like I earlier said, the outside world needs to know that you're a better person now.

Not by your words but by your actions. Do you get me? One of the ways you're going to live your spirituality is to forgive others.

Yeah… forgive them. You'll be doing more for yourself than you're doing for them.

Henri Nouwen wrote in "Bread for the Journey, a book of daily *meditations*,"

"To forgive another person from the heart is an act of liberation. We set that person free from the negative bonds that exist between us. We say, 'I no longer hold your offense against you.' But there is more. We also free ourselves from the burden of being the 'offended one.'…Forgiveness, therefore, liberates not only the other but also ourselves."

Forgiveness is another way of spiritual self-care. When you hold grudges against a person, that person gets a firm grip on your life.

You're probably going to think of that person even more than your lover or loved ones.

You'd just be going about your everyday business of the day or the hour, probably washing the clothes or something else, and you'd pause and be like;

"Stella, so you had the guts to try to steal Henry from me, huh? I swear I'll never forgive you for what you did. Never!"

You know that could even knock you off balance for the rest of your day, don't you? You'll probably start reminiscing on all that happened, the signs you saw and overlooked, the chats you read, etc. Then you'd start to cry and be gloomy for the rest of your day, not being able to achieve anything more meaningful than a head-splitting headache when you wake up the next day.

Stella has presumably forgiven herself and is living her best life. Maybe she came across a book like those, took the advice, forgave herself for the mistake, and moved on. But there you are, sulking all day for what's not worth it.

Try forgiveness today. You'll be surprised at how much better you'll feel than when you're bitter.

Perspective

Perspective, in simple words, means how we view or look at things, and it plays a vital role in all aspects of our lives. Perspective can also be seen as an approach to specific situations or problems. Two individuals can face the same problem, but how they approach it makes the most significant difference and determines if they'll come out of it wholly or damaged.

I had a friend back then in college. Collins. Back in our early years in college, he was always about studying just to make his papers, get a pass and move on to the next class until he graduated. It worked fine for him for the first two years until he struggled in his third year and had several spillover courses. He was so downcast that I was affected too. I remember speaking with him in an empty class. He did so well in his first two years, so I was forced to ask him what had happened to him.

He told me that he delayed studying till it was almost time for exams. He couldn't get everything into his head soon, and he had to pay for it.

Why did he stall? He didn't consider the knowledge essential enough for him to know. The only importance of the knowledge he acquired was for his answer script in the hall on exam day! So he was busy with the things he thought were more important till the time for his use of the knowledge came, and he couldn't get enough to help him scale through.

Now, my approach was quite different. Not too much of a bookworm, but I was big on knowing for knowing's sake, probably even for show off, and the knowledge I acquired extended beyond the exam papers. I wanted to have them because I wanted to have them, so I didn't wait till it was a week before examinations before I started studying; I created time to learn, so when it was almost time for exams, it was there. Probably with dust on it, it just required a little cleaning, and I was good to go.

Do you see we faced the same problem? But our approaches were different, and so were the results! That's the power of perspective. How one looks at a problem solves half the problem if we're to be honest.

Now that's for perspective on its own. What I'm going to talk about now is how we can use perspective as an effective tool to live our spirituality every day.

It's a simple principle. The quest for embracing our spirituality has no destination. It's a continuous path that has no place where we can stop, sigh and say;

"Oh, I finally made it!" And go for a drink or something to celebrate.

If you look at it like that and keep going hoping that one day you'll find a place where you can finally rest, you'll only get frustrated when you don't find any.

That's why perspective matters in this discussion. If you approach the subject of spirituality with a sense of an eternal journey, you already know that it gets better. I never stop, so you'll be glad instead of being frustrated and wondering when the journey will end with every step you take!

"Oh yeah! I got this part taken care of; What's next, what's next?" That's how it's going to be in your head.

Then you'll take a sip of wine because why not? You deserve it, don't you?

That's just how it works, girl. When you see this journey as eternal, you will see reasons to celebrate on the way. After all, if you wait till you arrive, you'll never celebrate because you'll never come.

How have you been seeing this journey? What has been your approach to this spirituality of a thing since you knew you needed it? Have you been seeing it as a journey with a destination or not? If you have, that's probably part of why you feel you're not going to make it work. Go back a little. Go back to the drawing board and advance slightly differently this time. Trust me; it will be one of the best decisions you'll ever make.

Release your Flowers

I mean, show your appreciation to others. What will it cost you if you show your sincere gratitude to others? Not a dollar. And how would you feel if someone fails to appreciate you for a job well done? Sad, right? Maybe angry too. So yeah, no matter who they are, total strangers or close friends and relatives? Give them their flowers, girl! It doesn't even cost you a flower to do that. Do you know that a little "thank you" will do just fine?

Do you have people working under you somewhere? Never forget to appreciate them and tell them how amazing they are, even if they're making mistakes. After correcting them, make sure you make them feel good before letting them go. If you were so mad that all you could do was yell at them, call them back and apologize for making them feel less of themselves when you're in a better frame of mind. Then go ahead to appreciate them for trying their best too. It would be best if you strived to make people smile and not be the source of their scorn. Respecting others will bring you a sense of fulfillment when you see the smile you've planted on a person's face.

Even when you're having a bad day, please don't make it an avenue to make it a bad day for other people who are also trying their best to live their best lives as well. You are never aware of what one act of unkindness can do to a person, so always try to keep it cool. It saves us a lot we're not even aware of.

So yeah! Release your flowers, woman. It doesn't hurt, nor does it harm. You'll even be in better shape than when you held it in.

Give

Just a four-letter word but even more powerful than we know it. I know plenty of us find it difficult to give other people what we've worked tirelessly for free, especially money, but there are other things to offer other than the money, you know?

What about your time? What about your talents? Even advice, knowledge, the list goes on and on. Give when you can and when you do, make sure you're giving with a genuine spirit and love.

Mother Teresa said in her book, ***A Simple Path,***

"It is not how much you do but how much love you put into the doing and sharing with others that is important."

So how are you giving today? Ask yourself. Are you sharing with a loving heart? Or you're giving grudgingly? If you give grudgingly, the receiver has nothing to lose. You're the one who's going to have to go through regrets. And regrets are not suitable for our souls; I hope you know that? So if you're going to give grudgingly, it's my advice that you don't provide. But don't just stay there to use it as an excuse not to share; learn how to give from a place of love and cultivate the act of giving. Because if you don't provide, you don't expect anyone to provide for you when you're in need. Now, this doesn't mean you should offer with the intention of getting something back from the receiver; that's quite shitty too. Just give freely, woman. It's an exercise that strengthens your spiritual muscles and gets you in good shape to fight off spiritual attacks. (Now, I don't mean principalities and powers, please.)

Alongside giving, also cultivate the act of receiving regardless of how small you think a gift is. That gift could mean the whole world to the giver, so you have to make sure you receive that gift wholeheartedly with gratitude as well.

This lets the giver know that he also has something to offer, no matter how small a gift is. The thought counts a lot of times.

Trust Your Guts

I'm not the only one who has heard that voice countless times telling us what to do in certain situations where we find ourselves in tight corners.

Every person, or should I say, a woman, has at one point or another in her life, heard the little voice saying;

"Hey, you! Go for it!" Or. "Why don't you calm down and see what happens."

Trust your guts, girl!

Maybe you don't know, but our guts are more accurate in telling us what to do in certain situations than our brains are. So instead of racking your brain and giving yourself sleepless nights, why don't you trust what your guts tell you to do? To me, it's a better option.

You must also understand that your guts do not speak to you every time. So when it does, please take it as a gift, trust it and follow it. It works damn fine. Believe me.

Learn and Practice Patience

You do not have to rush things in life. You've got to learn how to move one step at a time so you don't step too early into what you can't handle. Patience is indeed a virtue, and those who possess it to possess one of the greatest gifts one can ever ask for.

Do you need to rush into that relationship because you think he's got all you need in a man? Handsome, muscular, rich, caring, and all that? Do you even know if he loves you? You don't care because he's all you need in a man. But does he need you? You won't know all these when you're rushing.

So why don't you slow down a bit and take life one step at a time and see how things work out?

What about your everyday life? When you go to the shopping mall, you're in a situation where you've got to wait for a cashier or someone else to get something done for you? How do you behave? Do you scream at the top of your voice how "incompetent these people are?" I am not telling you not to lay a complaint when you're not satisfied with your service type. Nope. But then, how do you go about making your concern known? See? These things matter a lot in living your spirituality because this is you trying to manifest those positive virtues, patience being one of them. So, woman, what do you say?

Are you going to be patient? Or you're just going to let the essence of embracing spirituality come to nothing?

Express your Happiness!

No one gets an award for wearing a grimace and looking like a monster. If you're happy about something, why don't you show that you're happy, laugh, smile, come on! That's not cool! You might not be able to look happy when you're unfortunate, so why then would you not want to look happy when you're pleased. It's hard to believe, but people behave like that and find it amusing and troubling that people would sacrifice looking happy for... I don't even know what it is!

Pirtle, in *365 days of Happiness, says;*

"Laughing carries an energy of joy, silliness, playfulness, happiness, and fun,"

Going further, he said;

"When you laugh, you immediately shift to be and live in a 'high for life' frequency—and with that, you shift everything and everyone around you, too. If you choose to make laughing your default reaction, no matter what is happening for you, you will experience everything and everyone through your laughing filter."

Let me ask this question.

Do you think about your problems when you're laughing? I don't think I do. Do you see that laughing is very therapeutic?

Stop living in that illusion that wearing a straight face always makes one feared and respected.

First off, no one should fear you because you're not a serial killer.

Secondly, you will be respected for your behavior and not how you look.

One more thing.

"Take time to enjoy small, positive moments," says **Jamie Price,**

Little things and small moments matter a lot, some of which might even be more special than the big moments.

So as y'all black bold, beautiful women live spiritually, learn to cherish the small things and the small moments.

They hold much more than you think.

KEY POINTS

- By living our spirituality, we're building our spiritual energy as well.
- Spirituality is an internalized journey, but there's a need to show proof.
- There's always that thing that happens to us that we cannot explain.
- Let go of your mistakes and what others have done to you
- See spirituality as a journey and not a destination.
- It does you no good to hoard your compliments. Learn to appreciate other people.
- Give, and while you do, do so lovingly.

- When you're happy, show that you're happy. Laugh, smile, and be cheerful. To be genuinely happy is an opportunity you shouldn't take for granted.
- Listen to that inner voice, don't always rely on calculations.
- There's no need to rush things. It's slowly but surely.

CHAPTER SIX

PURGING YOURSELF OF EVIL ENERGY AND PEOPLE

"There are hundreds of paths up the mountain, all leading to the same place, so it doesn't matter which path you take. The only person wasting time is the one who runs around the mountain, telling everyone that his or her path is wrong."

– Hindu Proverb

We're going to be focusing our attention on the second sentence in the proverb above. It's essential to discuss the role that people around you play because in as much as the journey of spirituality is internalized, and like a personal journey, we shouldn't underestimate the power of other people in our lives don't you think so? Show me your friend, and I'll tell you who you are? Never gets old at all. So yeah, it's crucial the type of people you keep around you during this journey of spirituality. You have to consider what vibe they bring to the table and know whether to cut them off or let them stay.

What types of people do you need to have around during this delicate period of your life? And what are the kinds of people you wouldn't need to have around?

And again, what attitude do we need to put on during your journey? And what perspective do we not need to put on?

Let's take a walk through them, respectively.

"OVER-REALISTIC" PEOPLE

People like this always try to be rational in everything. Their favorite slang has to be;

"Let's be realistic here," or;

"It's just a coincidence."

For heaven's sake, not everything can be realistically explained or inquired into, for heaven's sake! And nothing is a coincidence! You've got to understand that, and anyone around you who doesn't want to understand that has to go. You don't have to make them your enemies, but they shouldn't have to hold so much importance in your life, or else it will put your spiritual journey in jeopardy.

These people love to question the existence of many abstract concepts, and as a woman who's chasing spirituality fiercely, that should be a turn-off. Of course, they will make fun of you, call you all sorts of names, call you uncool, blind, gullible, and many other forms of mockery. It shouldn't make you feel less of a person. That's one of the challenges you'll face in embarking on this journey. It means that you're on the right path!

How are these kinds of people going to make you distracted? You're an adult, and you know the difference between good and evil. Therefore, you should be responsible for your mishaps. Why blame the "influence" of other people for the cause of your misfortune?

These are questions that need to be answered before we move forward.

First off, don't you think it's better to abstain than stay amid people incompatible with your vision and beliefs? You might not be rewarded for "enduring through" the influence of other people in your life. Still, if you eventually fall prey to their schematics and they succeed in bending you over, it's not going to be a pleasant situation. Don't you think so?

So why test your perseverance with something as delicate as your spiritual journey? Any bad vibe or energy detected should be thrown off the window and with an immediate effect! A lot of things require that. Don't carry the burden on your shoulders; shake it off!

Now how are these kinds of people going to get you distracted?

These people are so dangerous that I don't even advise you to be careful with them; take to your heels and zoom off!

Why do I say they're dangerous? They're hazardous because they creep slowly up on you without your notice, and one thing you should know is that they don't give up easily. They don't even give up unless you give up on their company.

They don't give up because it's how they're built. They're neck-deep in trying to be the realistic and cool guy. They might not even be conscious of their influence. They're not going to call you to a corner and be like;

"Join us." No!

Your regular conversations and interactions with them are enough to do the job. Don't even try to argue; just let them go. Because one day, you'll try to see reasons with them and understand where they're coming from, and that's where it all starts. You're not going to be aware until you realize that you're already resonating with their takes on the subject. (I sincerely hope that's not already too late.) So wake up, woman! Especially when you're just starting your journey. That'll be too risky. Your foundation is still shaky, and it collapses with any negative impact.

So what's going to be your decision today? Are you going to sit back and listen to the women in the salon tell you that there's nothing beyond what we can see, feel, taste, smell, or hear? Or you're just going to ask them to get over your hair and get out of there immediately?

THE HYENAS

Now, who are the hyenas? They're the people who don't take anything seriously. Either deliberately or otherwise. These are the set of people that would likely call you funny names like the Virgin Mary, wife of Pope Francis; come on, name it all.

When you come to them with the subject, they want to make a joke so bad that they could sacrifice anything, I mean anything! Even as sacred as your spiritual journey, just for laughs. Pretty uncool, but you can't blame them; but one thing you can do is move out immediately! They don't deserve to be your audience for the time being. Let them go, or else they belittle something as delicate as your spirituality just for laughs.

THE SOCIAL MEDIA FREAKS

While embarking on this kind of journey, you don't want to be around people who seek validation from social media. That isn't healthy at all. Earlier in this book, I explained extensively that social media isn't your friend when working towards embracing your spirituality. So why be in the midst of people who live there and derive their values from unimportant things. That won't be smart. They're going to import those values as they live by them, and that's how their way of life will slowly influence you.

Under normal circumstances, you wouldn't even want to be with people that rely solely on social media for their values.

This is because social media is full of double standards. There's no real life in social media if we're to be completely honest. So when you notice girls, you roll with always freak out for the gram; that's a red flag. Run as fast as you can and pursue your spirituality more conveniently. There are already a lot of problems to face, so why add to it by wanting to fit in? Think again, woman!

BAG CHASERS

Bag chasers? Ridiculous! How the hell did I come up with a heading like that? Haha! I can't stop laughing, man! Outrageous! Well, that's for that; let's get back to business ASAP!

So who are the bag chasers? Bag chasers are the guys that are always after the money.

I know you should be expecting a "don't-get-me-wrong" next. Because why not? It would help if you didn't get me wrong here; money is a critical factor to be considered to live a comfortable life. Poverty should never be an option. But then, when you're always all about the money, not giving attention to other essential aspects of your life like your spirit that will be a lot for you to handle. Imagine having a lot of money and still not being fulfilled.

While you'd be doing great on the outside, you'd be dying on the inside because you failed to recognize the importance of your spiritual journey.

If you surround yourself with people like that, people who don't want to try to strike a balance and always want to be out there making the cash, you'll be distracted big time. Because while you're trying to bring up the issue of spirituality, they're always going to be there to shut you out and bring in some excuse that "makes a lot of sense." Because yeah, it seemingly does make a lot of sense to make money and be able to take care of yourself and your family and not go around begging on the streets. It'll be easier to see reasons to dump your spiritual journey and chase the bag entirely with the gang. After all, is spirituality going to put food on the table? Or put a roof over the head? Or put my skin under cotton? Not! But then, money still wouldn't be able to solve the problems that come with neglecting the pursuit of your spirituality.

Do you see why you should strike a balance and be around the people willing to strike a balance?

Money is good, damn good! But it isn't everything, and you have to understand that.

CONFUSED PEOPLE

I'm sorry to say this, but I've got to say it. Avoid confused people like the plague, especially when you're just setting out early in the journey. Trust me; they'll do more harm than good. They're going to be here today and there tomorrow, and you're going to be confused like they are too. You might even question your journey and be like;

"Am I even doing this right? Or should I be doing this at all?" Those are tough questions to ask yourself when you're on a spiritual journey. Because answers will find you, and if the wrong one sees you, that's not healthy. You're going to lose your guard, and if you don't have anyone to put you back on track, you're going to fall out and start thinking that this spirituality of a thing doesn't even work! But then you're the one to blame. That's a hilarious situation to be in, and avoid problems like that; you've got to avoid mingling with confused people. They're bad vibes, I'm afraid.

JUDGES

By choosing to run this race, you're choosing to do away with certain vices, and you don't want to be around people who are experts in the field. One of those things you're going to have to do away with is being judgmental, so you wouldn't want to be around people who are judging others.

Let's not even talk about the fact that you might be the next to be placed in the dock as soon as you leave the table because it doesn't matter what they say about you. The subject of discourse here is solely based on how these people will influence you if you don't have a firm stand on the grounds of spirituality.

You can't be in the midst of people who judge and not judge yourself. That's one of the things spirituality preaches against, which will make you a hypocrite.

Hypocrites are also another set of people you should avoid at all costs. They claim to be spiritual when they're not close, so what's the use? Come out clean rather than hide in the guise of chasing spirituality when you're doing the total opposite. If any of you women finds yourself among such people, its high time you saw an exit route; otherwise, you will be like them. And trust me, you're not lying to anybody else, you're only lying to yourself, and that'll be to your detriment.

PEOPLE WHO ALWAYS GIVE YOU THE THUMBS UP

I wish I could get a fancier heading for this. But I'd console myself with the fact that I've been calm all through. So this won't be too much of a problem.

People like this are slow killers. They see you walking into a fire, and when you look back at them, they give you a thumbs up and be like;

"You're doing great, girl!"

"Go, girl."

"Yasss, queen."

They say so many things, woman, don't be careful with them, walk them out of your life!

Do you know what's funny? When you get burnt, they will be the same people to laugh at you and make a big fuss out of your mistake. That's going to sting so much, you know? So this is what you need to do.

Be with the people who tell you the plain truth, unfiltered. Do away with the people who always give you approval. You can't always be correct. So when all they do is tell you you're doing great, even when you know that you're walking into the deep blue sea, run as fast as you can away from them. They don't mean good at all. They're deliberately toxic and don't want you to be the person you strive to be. Make sure you cut them off without hesitation!

It could also mean that these people don't care for you enough to take their time to scrutinize your actions, so they tell you to go ahead, not caring about what the consequences will be. These people are not fit for your journey. Take them out immediately without any explanation. They don't even care, so good for you both.

For a while, I've been all about the different kinds of people we should avoid in this sacred journey of spirituality. But then, I won't forget to mention that there are certain attitudes I would consider lousy energy and wouldn't be of much help to your journey to embracing your spirituality. I said I would talk about them earlier, so let's get to it before I wrap up this chapter.

DOUBT

This is undoubtedly bad vibes. Don't ever doubt your journey or your ability to take the trip. That would only allow the people I mentioned above to take control and ruin your journey, and you may not even know it.

When you doubt your journey, you're calling to question its truth. And when you do that for long, you become discouraged and no more interested in the journey. Don't let that doubt take over you, girl. Beat it and make me proud. You know the interesting thing, these feelings come in subtlety and slowly eat you until you're all finished and can't do anything anymore. If you have gone a little bit far in your journey, it'll draw you back to square one, and trust me, starting all over will probably be the most challenging thing you'll ever do.

So clear that doubt now, woman. Some people have started the journey before you. Look at them. If they can do it, you certainly can do it too. So don't you ever think you can't.

REGRET

People always remind themselves of all their mistakes and choose to live in them, which is wrong! That's evil energy! Do you notice that I said, "For some reason"? You should have. Now I say that because there's no reason people regret it most of the time. Crazy.

It just comes and sweeps you off your feet, taking you back to the times when you made a mistake that cost you something and makes you sulk over it when the only thing you should do is get better and try not to make the same mistake anymore.

You might even be over it and moving on with your life and your journey, but then your mind wants to flashback and relives that terrible memory of when you messed up and had to pay for it. It slows your trip and can even create room for doubt. Because if I could make such a mistake back then, should I even be here in the first place? That's how doubt sets in. You can see how one thing leads to the other and then hinders you from making meaningful strides in the journey of your spirituality. Don't you ever give room for regrets? Like I'll always say, they're a bad vibe!

IMPOSTOR SYNDROME

You get this feeling when you think you don't have what it takes to be someone or do something. And when you get something important done, you attribute it to luck or something else but yourself. It's closely associated with doubt, but there are distinctions. While primary factors like regret fuel doubt, impostor syndrome is caused by remote factors, which can even be from childhood.

Maybe your parents pressured you to do well in school, compared you to your sibling(s), were controlling or overprotective, emphasized your natural intelligence, and sharply criticized your mistakes.

You start to feel like you can't measure up and strive too hard, only to get burned out and feel more frustrated and still not fulfilled or satisfied.

The truth is, you need to give yourself credit sometimes. Yeah! It's good for your mental health. You have to give yourself a thumbs up sometimes and be like, I did it, and I did it exceedingly well! That will make you pumped up for what the next big challenge is. But then impostor syndrome prevents you from taking credits. It tells you that you're not worth the hype; even when people around you tell you that you're doing a great job, you're still not satisfied. That's a significant hindrance to one's spiritual journey.

How do we overcome impostor syndrome?

This topic will be like a bonus one here because this topic is broad. So take this as a gift from me to you, my wonderful black beautiful woman, because you deserve it and even more.

I'm going to walk you through some steps to overcome this phenomenon, and I hope you put them to practice because they'll help a lot, trust me.

Notice the Signs

Before you tackle a problem, you've got to know that you have the problem first. You can't possibly fix what you don't know anything about, so you've got to make sure you know that, yeah... "Something's got to be wrong with me."

Here are a few signs you need to look out for.

- You find it hard to accept praise even when it's well deserved.

- Even when you were armed to the teeth and prepared well, you feel like you "got lucky."

- You're overly scared of failure. The thought alone makes you sick

- You're a hundred percent convinced that you're not enough.

- You avoid openly taking credit for your achievements because people will see it as proud and saucy.

These are a few signs you should always look out for. If you notice these signs, you might be running a risk of having imposter syndrome.

Distinguish Between Humility and Fear

You have to recognize that it is one thing to take credit for your milestones and accomplishments and another thing to be overcome with fear due to taking credit for them.

Being scared is normal, but then you have to bring a balance. It's possible to take credit without making it seem like you're proud. You know that's one of the signs. Scared of people thinking that you're obnoxious when you voice out your achievements. But I'll tell you something just like one **Seth Godin** wrote;

"Humility and worthiness have nothing to do with defending our territory. We don't have to feel like a fraud to be gracious, open or humble."

I urge you to reflect on those words.

Release the Pressure

Be kind to yourself and stop questioning your ability to get things done. It mounts a lot of pressure on us and slowly, mentally destroys us. Impostor syndrome is not like a skin disease or something that outwardly shows. It manifests itself as a voice in your head, feeding you with negative comments.

So be kind to yourself, learn, and practice positive self-talk.

It helps you build the courage to do more extraordinary things.

Another thing you can do is to capture those moments when the negative thoughts filter in, then counter them by thinking positively. For example, when you find yourself feeling like, "oh, I ain't worthy of this," or "I just got lucky," counter those thoughts by taking your mind back to how you made it happen, the steps you took, the sleepless nights, anything at all that reminds you of how hard you worked for what you got. It goes a very long way to help battle impostor syndrome.

Document Your Wins

When faced with impostor syndrome, you find it hard to understand how much you did and what role you played in your achievements. Then you begin to attribute your wins to fate, luck or even the hard work of others.

So this is what you need to do that'll help as well.

Have a journal to document your accomplishments and what you did to make them happen. It'll be a very good reminder in the future when negative thoughts start filtering in.

Imagine you have a book you could quickly turn to remind yourself how much of a monster you are! You could call it your "Book of Success." You might even want to go through it every day. It will make you realize that you can do more than that, and it's a plus for you!

Let It Work For You

I will be the wrong person and a liar if I tell you that one can completely get rid of the impostor syndrome because you can't possibly do that. But what you can do is embrace it, stop it from hindering your success and use it to forge your success!

Many successful people said they've battled and are still battling the condition.

Actor Don Cheadle said this about himself;

"...All I can see is everything I'm doing wrong that is a sham and a fraud."

But then, if it didn't stop them from achieving the heights they've gotten to, then it definitely wouldn't stop a strong black woman from achieving what they wish to achieve.

With this, I've come to the end of my little lecture on impostor syndrome as a gift to my wonderful black woman. Learn to cope with this phenomenon and be strengthened to keep moving on in the journey of your spirituality.

I believe in you, ladies, and you should believe in yourself too!

KEY POINTS

- As much as the journey of spirituality is personal, other people also play a massive role for the better.

- You don't need to be too realistic in the pursuit of spirituality

- Don't hesitate to let go of people whose reasoning does not resonate with yours. Especially as someone new to the race.

- Most of the time, people's influence on each other is not a conscious effort.

- Spirituality should not be what you joke with. There are other things to laugh about.

- Money can't solve spiritual issues.

- You're not always right; avoid people who don't tell you the truth.

- Never give room for doubt in the journey of spirituality.

- In this journey, whatever mistake you made in the past stays in the past. The only use of errors is to teach lessons.

- Taking credits for your wins doesn't make you arrogant. Learn to acknowledge that you're good enough and worthy of every accomplishment you've worked hard for.

CHAPTER SEVEN

WHAT'S THE CONNECTION?

RELATING SEXUALITY TO SPIRITUALITY

"When we touch the place in our lives where sexuality and spirituality come together, we touch our wholeness and the fullness of our power and, at the same time, our connection with a power larger than ourselves."

Judith Plaskow

Before I begin this lengthy talk about sexuality and spirituality, I have a story to tell you, my dear black woman, and I hope you stay with me till the end. I don't usually share this story with people because it's not entirely about me, and even though I've been permitted to share it, I sometimes feel terrible about it due to some of my past actions. However, I would gladly tell you because I am committed to seeing you grow spiritually. So shall we?

I had a girlfriend whose name I'd like to withhold seven years ago and instead call Zee. After numerous flings and a handful of relationships I had been in, I decided I was in love. I could feel it. I was sure that I loved Zee, and it wasn't even a question of whether she loved me. She even loved me more than I did, and at times it was scary, but I took solace in the fact that it didn't matter so much. It was precisely a year before I popped the question, and she happily said yes to me. Until then, I didn't know much about her family or anything about her. All I knew, she told me, and she told me what she wanted me to know.

Skip to a month to our wedding, and Zee changed overnight. LITERALLY. Especially in the area of intimacy. It was like she felt disgusted by every touch of mine, and I started having feelings of suspicion. My suspicions were proven accurate, but I couldn't even be angry. I was dumbfounded. Zee was bi. Yeah, she was bisexual.

My initial reaction was, "What the FUCK?"

I didn't hesitate to let her know I was utterly upset because she not only cheated on me but kept her sexuality a secret for the one year and four months we were together. Without waiting for an explanation, I left her house and cut off all communications with her.

When I think about my reaction, all I want to do is hope that the ground splits into two and eats me whole because it's downright embarrassing. Two months later, I began to ask myself why I didn't wait to hear her side of the story, why I judged her so quickly after claiming to love her, why I did this, and why I did that.

It became unbearable at some point, so I placed a call to her, and surprisingly, she was willing to talk to me. We met at our favorite café to talk about what exactly happened. I could tell she was doing fine without me, probably with her girlfriend; I would never know, whereas I looked like shit.

So Zee told me that she felt more love for me than she had felt for anyone she ever dated and that everything changed a day after I proposed. A hot lesbian chic on the block that is only interested in 'straight' girls decided to get Zee.

Zee told me something vital to sexuality, which I would be talking about extensively; thank you very much. She said it was all confusing for her, getting to know her sexuality, but with the coming of her new lover, everything seemed just right. She had struggled with knowing her proper sexual orientation since childhood and while being heterosexual felt good, being bisexual made her feel the freedom she never felt. That was all I needed to know.

I felt it was me for months – that I was the one at fault. Maybe I wasn't doing it right, maybe my sex game wasn't as good, but it was all Zee. It had all been her. While I felt relieved, I could never get over the fact that I judged and almost hated her for embracing her true sexuality.

Now, connecting sexuality and spirituality looks pretty unusual, absurd even. A lot of people look at sexuality from the physiologist's lens. They're only about the physical aspects, the pleasure, and the rest. But the truth remains – a very subtle truth, though – getting in touch with your spirituality makes life a lot easier to live because you've found what works for you.

You're going to love your life that way regardless of what anyone says, provided that you're not propagating anything evil or spiteful or even something you wouldn't want anyone to do to you. If embracing spirituality makes one live life on more simple terms, imagine applying that spirituality you've adopted to other aspects of your life; Sexuality being one aspect of your spirituality is needed.

Okay, okay, it seems I'm already boarding the boat and leaving you at sea, so I'm going to take this slow, much slower, and more detailed than the rest of the topics I've talked about because of how delicate this topic is. This concept of sexuality isn't discussed every time, and even when it is tabled, not enough justice is usually done to it. You must adequately understand this because it's a prerequisite to accessing your full girl power, my dear black woman.

When the topic of sexuality pops up in our faces, what comes to most minds is how we understand our bodies about sex and relationships. Merriam Webster's dictionary defines sexuality as "the quality or state of being sexual: the condition of having sex; sexual activity; expression of sexual receptivity or interest especially when excessive," and the Oxfords English Dictionary backs it up by defining it as "the feelings and activities connected with a person's sexual desires."

These definitions are exciting and helpful in the slightest sense, but what if I told you there was more to sexuality than "the state of being sexual" or "the feelings and activities connected with a person's sexual desires?"

Sexuality is one of the fundamental forces behind people's thoughts, behaviors, and feelings. It encompasses how procreation occurs and talks about one's psychological and sociological beliefs about sex. Sexuality is regulated by various parts of the brain, which shape the body and mind towards seeking pleasure. As much as practicing is essential to acknowledge your sexuality fully, just the slightest thoughts and fantasies can be considered ways of experiencing and expressing your sexuality?

There's nothing to be ashamed of about sexuality, as it is a significant part of being human. The entirety of sexuality is about sex, sexual orientation, reproduction, gender identity, and pleasure, so it is not out of place that either of these keywords frequently appears when we talk about a topic as exciting and delicate as this.

Overview of Sex

Sex pushes us to do many things, making babies one of the significant reasons which used to be the primary reason people indulged in sex back in the day. Sex makes us feel perfect if you know what I mean; it gives us pleasure, and you may even say our bodies are built for sex.

There are many health benefits of sex, and I'll list a few;

- Helps for a more robust immune system.

- Allows for effective pain relief.

- Helps take away signs of depression.

- A great confidence booster.

- Strengthens your muscles, etcetera.

There are a lot of factors that can influence our sexual experience. These include age, gender, mass media, race, marital status, parents, cultures, religious and spiritual beliefs, etc.

Some significant factors such as cultural and religious beliefs can influence how a person views sex and sexuality and reacts to these concepts. These factors can either cause shame or uplift an individual, depending on how the individual reacts to them.

Sexual trauma is another factor that can influence our sexual experience. Some people who have been raped or assaulted may go through depression and feel numb or hateful towards sex.

Sex can be used interchangeably with sexuality, but it is just one part of sexuality.

A Brief History of Human Sexuality

The history of human sexuality goes way back over 200,000 years ago. It's almost as old as human history. Just as creativity, writing, and speech can be traced more than a hundred thousand years back, sex can also be outlined. Artifacts recovered from ancient cultures, when examined, have been recorded to be fertility totems. An ancient text referred to as the Kama Sutra, which dates from 400 BCE to 200 CE, is an Indian text that talks about sexuality, pleasure, and emotional fulfillment. It's like a manual for sex and a guide to sexuality that discusses the nature of love, finding love, maintaining your relationship, and everything related to love and sex. Just like the Kama Sutra, the Qur'an, Bible, and Torah also give rules and advice as well as tell stories about sex since antiquity.

The thing is, sex has been around from the time of conception, but scientists only started investigating sex around the '80s until now. In 1837, Alexander Jean Baptiste Parsnt-Duchatelet published a 1830s study on prostitutes in Paris. The prostitutes were about 3,558 and were registered. That study was the first work of modern sex research.

A method of research known as the case study method came about during the 190s, and it was said to be employed by scientists in the investigations of sex. Some of the best case studies were carried out by Sigmund Freud, an Australian Neurologist who founded psychoanalysis. He is believed to be the first scientist to set a connection between sex and healthy development in humans. He believed human beings are sexual and refuted the widespread belief that children cannot have sexual feelings. This redefinition of sexuality and the inclusion of children in it led him to formulate the term "Oedipus complex." He also argued that developing a person's personality from childhood passes through five psychosexual stages: oral, anal, phallic, latency, and genital stages. There's an expression of libido during these stages and across parts of the body.

Henry Havelock Ellis, an English physician who studied human sexuality, also published works about human sexuality. Some of his famous works are on transgender people and how they are different from homosexuals. He advocated for women's education on human sexuality and believed that if women were given a chance, they would choose better sexual partners.

I can't end this talk on the brief history of human sexuality without mentioning the father of human sexuality research, Alfred Charles Kinsey, an American biologist and the founder of the Institute for Sex Research located at Indiana University. Some of his books are Sexual Behavior in the Human Male (1948) and Sexual Behavior in the Human Female (1953). He was initially an expert on wasps before he redirected his course of study to humans.

He is widely known as the first significant figure in American sexology whose research spurred sexologists to explore human sexuality. Not only did he encourage sexologists with his work, but he argued against the popular notion that women were generally not sexual beings. So we have this science god to thank amongst many others when studying female sexuality.

What is a Woman's Sexuality?

I stated earlier that sexuality is one of the fundamental forces behind people's thoughts, behaviors, and feelings. It encompasses how procreation occurs and talks about one's psychological and sociological beliefs about sex. Sexuality is about accepting who you are and all that you've experienced. It's about exploring and taking total control of your own body. A woman who's confident in her sexuality is a strong woman who can define pleasure on her terms and not bend to the whims of others.

Sexuality is regulated by various parts of the brain, which shape the body and mind towards seeking pleasure. The entirety of sexuality is about sex, sexual orientation, reproduction, gender identity, and fun.

Now, my beautiful black woman, a woman's sexuality is about different behaviors exhibited by women. These behaviors include the sexual orientation and behavior of women. Sexuality is influenced by several factors such as psychological, cultural, religious, legal, spiritual, and a host of other factors.

Talking about the cultural factor, the arts of that particular culture shows a significant part of what society thinks about human sexuality. It includes both the covert and overt aspects of female sexuality and behavior.

A legal factor could present boundaries and limits to sexual behavior, stating what is and isn't allowed in society. Female sexuality, like sexuality in general, cuts across all regions of the world and is constantly changing.

You might be born with particular sexuality as a woman. Still, with your exposure to your environment, your religious beliefs, and others, you find that you've evolved and picked up another sexuality. As a woman, you might feel a great urge towards sex, but you may not feel anything sometimes. It's all part of being a woman.

With this, we can now delve into the topic thoroughly. I hope your attention is still with me because I'm about to answer the bugging question, what is a woman's sexuality?

It's all we've been saying about sexuality. When a woman can feel a certain way, have a sensual reaction, and be attracted to people, we're talking about her sexuality. It's also about a female choosing who she has sex with. Finding people to who you're attracted in a sexual, emotional, or physical way is a part of your sexuality. It is one thing to find out your true sexuality and another to explore and express it. Ways in which you can explore and express your sexuality can be found in things like fantasizing about a person or sex, masturbating, kissing, sexual dreams, and penetrative or oral sex.

Sexual Development

Infants do not see the opposite sex as the opposite sex. They know if this person is my friend, then they are. There's no stress over which gender they belong to. You could kiss a baby, and they would giggle and not feel any sexual tension between you two because they're simply infants, and sexual hormones in them have not yet been released.

In early childhood, usually starting from age 3, a child begins to become aware of the other gender and its gender.

Biological research suggests that androgens play a definite role in deciding which gender gets the sensitive part and specific behaviors.

During the adolescent stages, significant sexual developments occur in the human body, and it is in this stage we reach puberty. Puberty is a phase of transition during which significant effects of sexuality occur. Puberty, as we know, is the peak of sexual maturity—the period where a male or female is capable of reproduction.

Puberty in Girls

Puberty in girls begins at around ages 8 and 13 years old. It is a period where a child's body begins to mature as they grow toward adulthood. The first sign is that their breasts develop and grow more significant for girls. Other signs of puberty in girls are body hair growth, vaginal discharge, menstruation, wider hips, increase in height, etcetera.

These changes all work towards ensuring the ability to reproduce in a woman. The changes can be internal or external. Puberty starts in the brain. It begins in the parts of the brain that oversee bodily functions such as blood pressure, temperature, and heart rate. The brain also produces chemicals that travel to the bloodstream through specific organs. These sex organs are, in turn, stimulated to release sex hormones.

A female hormone called estrogen is released by a girl's ovaries when stimulated. It is this hormone that causes the changes in girls associated with puberty. The balance of progesterone and estrogen causes menstruation.

Sexual feelings usually develop when a female hits puberty or at an adolescent stage. We very well know what comes with sexual feelings; the attraction to either male or female, sexual dreams, masturbation, and the likes. It's all a normal phase required for the growth of the female.

The female brain constantly develops up till the age of 25, and there are a lot of changes that come with it. This development can affect our abilities to make decisions, but we should strive to make the right decisions that will always make us feel safe.

Control Over Women's Sexuality; Double Standards

I went to several places and countries to get first-hand

information and people's opinions about sexuality regarding my research on this topic. While many were willing to talk openly about it, numerous others saw it as shameful and went as far as shuddering at the mention of this topic. You can guess that women took up a large chunk of the numbers among these numerous people.

I find that there are a lot of double standards held by society when it comes to sexuality. A glaring example is how culture encourages a man to have free sexuality while a woman is told to deny hers. A man is applauded for having multiple sexual partners, and a woman scorned, spat on, and called all sorts of names for doing the same thing a man would do concerning sexual freedom. Men are cheered on when they indulge in pre-marital sex, while girls are stigmatized and shunned for doing the same.

Many attempts have been made in the past and present to nullify women's sexuality completely. "It's a man's world" and, as such, desire that women be trodden upon. Mastering your sexuality is a key to unlocking the treasure chests inside you, my dear black woman, so strive hard, by all means, to do so.

Even in most cultural practices, FGM, which is short for Female Genital Mutilation, continues today, and it's highly appalling, the least to say. I want to take a moment to applaud everyone who is constantly fighting against this barbaric practice and hope that someday, it will be outlawed in all nations.

Besides FGM, several methods have been employed to control female sexuality, such as honor killings, shame, wrong teachings, and fear.

Honor Killings

An honor killing or shame killing is the murder of an individual who could be an outsider or part of a family by someone desperate to protect their so-called dignity and honor. Most honor killings are nurtured in a misogynistic society as they are usually targeted at women. A woman can be killed for critical reasons such as speaking out as a victim of sexual assaults, refusing to succumb to an arranged marriage, committing adultery, inappropriate dressings, or seeking a divorce – even in cases of an abusive husband.

Honor killings are prevalent in Pakistan, Bangladesh, India, and Indonesia, with these countries having the top record of honor killings.

Shame

Most women are made to go through terrible experiences in their life that leave them with feelings of shame regarding their gender. Revealing cleavage in the media is becoming a norm, and women who engage in such acts are applauded and accepted by the society that calls them sexy. However, the reverse is the case for nursing mothers shamed for publicly breastfeeding their children. It even goes as far as kicking them out of public places for such a simple act of love that society deemed inappropriate. It's tiring because this is only the tip of the iceberg regarding the numerous times' women have been shamed.

It even goes as far as society condemning women to talk about indulging in masturbation. Oh yes. A historical device known as the chastity belt was used to control female sexual behavior. It's like a piece of clothing with a lock designed for and worn by women to prevent sexual intercourse. As the name implies, they were worn to protect women's virtue and avoid any unauthorized male or masturbation by the woman who wore them. I cannot imagine the level of shame such women had to face.

Wrong Teachings

The propaganda against women's sexuality is pushed when society decides to lie to the female child and give wrong teachings instead. Girls are taught to hate sex and masturbation. They are told that they're all acts of sin and should wait until marriage, whereas a boy who hasn't masturbated is frowned upon. Society encourages boys but not girls to explore their sexuality, masturbate, take charge of what they want, and discover pleasure, but neglects that women are humans and should be given the freedom to explore their bodies.

Fear

Do you know that doctors examine the hymen of a woman to check if she has had sex or not? Girls are told that if the hymen isn't intact, they're no longer virgins and that it's a taboo. So out of fear, girls recoil and are afraid to participate in their best sports so their hymen wouldn't break, but what if I told you that hymens do not break? Yes, my beautiful black woman! Hymens can stretch and cause a small tear, but it certainly doesn't break. This is why you need to be in charge of your sexuality and know who you are. You are a queen and shouldn't let anyone tell you otherwise. You are powerful, and no one should be allowed to talk you down!

While the list is endless, I do not wish to dwell on the negative but to attend to the negative and turn it into positivity. With so much conviction in my heart and all my research on women's sexuality, I do believe if you walk with me completely, not faltering or doubting, you'll be able to know, embrace and fully express your sexuality. Oh, and don't worry, you'll see how your sexuality can affect your spirituality. Sit tight, beautiful black woman. It's going to be a fun ride!

IDENTITY DEVELOPMENT

SEXUAL IDENTITY, SEXUAL ORIENTATION, AND SEXUAL BEHAVIOR

Sexual Identity

Sexual identity has to do with how a person thinks of themselves to whom they're sexually or romantically attracted. It can also be referred to as sexual orientation identity, a term for when people choose to identify or choose not to identify with a particular type of sexual orientation.

This term is related to sexual orientation and sexual behavior, but they can be differentiated. I'll give distinct definitions first and move ahead to talk some more about each of them.

Sexual identity is what a person thinks or conceives of his or herself sexually,

Sexual behavior refers to the sexual acts which an individual engages in, an

Sexual orientation, a part of sexual identity, is about how you feel sexually towards others. It entails your sexual attraction towards the opposite gender, the same gender, both genders, and even none at all.

So if I believe that I'm heterosexual and affirm that I am, that's my sexual identity. If I feel only attracted and wish to have sex with the opposite gender, my sexual orientation. Then if I have sex with the opposite gender, no matter the race or ethnicity, that's my sexual behavior.

You see, they're alike but different. Now we can go back to sexual identity.

Developing a stable consciousness of yourself and your role in society is an excellent sign that you're experiencing a healthy development as an adolescent. For an individual to be fully prepared for intimacy, he needs to have a strong sense of their sexuality. Ways in ways adolescents develop sexually include role-play and experiment.

Knowing one's sexuality is needed for intimacy and having sexual intercourse. Still, your sexual identity can change over time and diverge from the known sexual behavior, orientation, or biological sex.

Amongst sexual orientation and sexual behavior, sexual identity is more closely related to sexual behavior. For instance, homosexual and bisexual men and women are more prone to having sex with someone of the same sex, in contrast to a lesser percent of men and women who had attractions to people of the same sex. This is because more and more people understand who they are and what they want and going for it. Gender and sex are essential parts of a person's identity, but they do not necessarily tell us about their sexual orientation.

Sexual Behavior

Sexual behavior, human sexual practice, or human sexual activity has to do with how individuals express their sexuality. It encompasses the sexual acts people engage in concerning their sexuality. These sexual acts range from masturbation, sexual intercourse, oral sex, etcetera. Some cultures and religions frown upon sexual activities outside of marriage, while some sexual activities such as sexual assault and rape are considered illegal universally.

Sexual Orientation

As stated earlier, sexual orientation is about how you feel sexually towards other people. For further explanation, it can be defined as the ability of someone to sexually arouse the interest of another person or the sexual attractions one can feel towards another person.

Sexual orientation can be classified into the following:

Heterosexuality

Heterosexuals are commonly called 'straight' people. Heterosexuality is a type of orientation where a person feels attracted to another person or persons of the opposite sex. This type of identity group is the largest sexual identity group globally.

Homosexuality

This is a type of sexuality where a person is attracted only to the same sex. So a man can be attracted to another man, and he's called a homosexual man or gay, while a woman can be attracted to another woman, and she's tagged a homosexual woman, lesbian, or less frequent times, gay.

Bisexuality

As the name implies, this type of sexuality is a person attracted to both male and female genders. People who embrace this identity are called bisexuals. They do not necessarily need to like both genders equally. It all boils down to the fact that they can choose to have sex with any gender, despite seemingly being committed to one gender.

Pansexuality

When people are sexually attracted to others regardless of their gender identity or sex, you can say they are pansexuals. Pansexuality has to do with gender-blindness. Pansexuals focus on other reasons and not gender to be romantically or sexually attracted to others. It can be considered a type of bisexuality.

Asexuality

Asexuality is different from the rest. Asexuals lack sexual attraction to other people. Their interest in sexual activities is usually absent or, if present at all, minimal. It is important to note that asexuality is entirely different from abstention and celibacy.

Polysexuality

This is sometimes used interchangeably with bisexuality. It's not precisely different as it encompasses various types of sexuality. A person is usually sexually attracted to many people but not all genders.

Unlabeled Sexuality

This is when an individual chooses not to fall under any sexual identity. Individuals can refuse to label their sexuality because it makes them feel put in a 'box' or unsure of their sexuality. I may not like the labels that come with a specific type of sexuality and wish to feel free, so I'd choose to be unlabeled. Most people who decide to be unlabeled prefer to be sexually attracted to a person and not their gender.

Some women identify as unlabeled because of their uncertainty about the types of relationships they might later choose to have. I could refuse to label my sexuality because I want to feel free. I wouldn't want to feel compelled or forced to be attracted to someone my sexual identity says I should. Do you understand, my beautiful black woman?

Overall, we're constantly developing, so it's okay for your sexuality to change. It may change, it may not, but most importantly, I need you to understand that it's magnificent to feel the way you think, and you don't have to judge yourself for it.

Gender Identity

Gender identity is related to sexuality in a way. It's defined as the conception of yourself. So as a woman, if you choose to identify or be called a woman, then no one can call you a man. And if, as a woman, you decide to be called a man, do things that men do and act like a man to identify with the gender, you would be called a man. The same goes for men, it looks complex, but it's simple.

A person born as a female can choose to identify as a man, and when they have sexual relations with a woman, they can be called a heterosexual. Still, if a female who identifies as a male chooses to have sexual intercourse with a male, they're gay.

As children, we were taught about the cultural norms of masculinity and femininity. It was common for a girl to have long hair or long dresses, and we've come to terms with it. Some cultures even attribute the building of houses to men, while cooking was a woman's job. But the thing is, culture changes over time; hence the beliefs about gender can also change. Formally, pink was associated with femininity, while blue was for boys. About a century ago, there was a revolution, and these same cultures changed their ideas and had baby boys wearing pink clothing and girls in blue.

A typical attitude towards people who identify outside the gender they see as 'normal,' such as – a boy identifying as a boy and a girl identifying as a girl or the 'common' sexual orientation, which is heterosexuality – is that of hostility and discrimination. Members of the LGBTQ+ community are treated in the most hostile manners, and some are even imprisoned and given different sentences in countries where gay activities aren't legalized.

As a part of our spiritual growth and a journey to loving ourselves and each other, discrimination against someone based on their sexual orientation or behavior and gender identity should not be acceptable. For a better society and humanity to move forward, it is only proper to show love to everyone around us and accept everyone, no matter their choices. I don't see why you should hate or discriminate against anyone for choosing to love or have sex with someone of a different gender when they are in no way causing harm to you. My beautiful black woman, what do you think?

Types of Gender Identities.

Cisgender

Like heterosexuality, cisgender seems to be the leading gender identity. It refers to people who still identify with their birth sex. So if you were born as a female at birth and choose to remain with that identity, you're a cisgender woman.

Transgender

It's an umbrella term for people who transition through medical assistance from their birth sex to their desired sex. They're more than just the trans men and trans women but include non-binary or gender queer. On a broad scale, transgender people can be called cross-dressers.

Bigender

Bigender is a term relating to a person who has a combination of two genders. They have just two genders, masculine and feminine.

Omnigender

This refers to seeing all genders as the same and not discriminating against one from the other. An omnigender person can possess only one gender but can easily pass it off for another.

Agender

People under this identity are indifferent toward identifying with any gender. At times, they do not have any gender at all. Agender can also be called genderless, neutral gender, null-gender, or neutrinos. Androgyne is a synonymous word that is slightly different from the other words. It is a mixture of masculinity and femininity, and they have the characteristics of both a man and a woman's behaviors.

Butch

This is a term used in lesbianism. It's associated with a lesbian who expresses more masculinity. Femme is the opposite of Butch. A lesbian who represents more femininity is called a femme. Butch can be said as a type of gender identity, as most homosexuals are familiar with this.

Gender Expansive

It's an umbrella term recognized by the LGBTQIA for persons who choose to push past definitions of gender held by their culture. They express their sexuality outside of what their culture would expect. Transgender people are part of gender-expansive.

Genderfluid

A person who identifies as genderfluid doesn't have a fixed expression of their identity. The person could feel masculine in a particular place at a specific time, but when they leave that environment, his identity changes to feminine, like a fluctuation.

Gender Outlaw

Like a fish out of water, a gender outlaw refuses to let society's definition of masculinity and femininity define them.

Genderqueer

Also called non-binary, genderqueer persons refuse to identify as either male or female. They do not classify under the gender binary but fit more under the transgender umbrella, although some genderqueer persons do not consider themselves transgender.

Masculine of Center

Let's call it boyishness. In the LGBTQ community, masculine of center (MOC) persons are lesbians or trans or bend more towards the masculinity line.

Polygender and Pangender

Persons in this identity group have multiple gender identities.

....

HOW SEXUALITY AFFECTS SPIRITUALITY

IS THERE A POSSIBILITY?

When I first came across this topic many years ago as a teenager, I was utterly perplexed and raised my eyebrows in wonder and confusion about how these concepts were connected. As an adult with many years of sexual and spiritual experience who's here to guide you, it gives me so much pleasure that I'm writing about this. I can't help but let a small smile creep up my lips because the concepts are entirely on fire.

Years ago, I made friends with a woman called Kira. We hardly see each other anymore because she moved recently after getting married, but I place a call to check up on her whenever I can. She does so, too. It's a mutual friendship.

When we first became friends, we listened to a podcast on spirituality that got us talking on a particular day, and I can still remember her words. "It's either sex or spirituality. They don't align."

I knew little about spirituality and sexuality back then, so I couldn't hold a solid argument. Kira had been brainwashed with the false narrative that she had to choose between sex and pursuing her spiritual life, and somehow she managed to convince me too. But it was only for a short while because I didn't believe in a thing such as spirituality. Now that I think about it, it's funny how convicted she was, and it's sad because, for a great deal of her life, she stuck to the spiritual part because, according to her, whenever she tried to merge both, they always repelled, like both sides of a magnet.

When I took a course on sexuality and spirituality, I learned that I needed affirmation—something to remind me that sexuality and spirituality went hand in hand. I went back to Kira and asked if she was still convicted. This time, her reply was utterly different. She had switched from spirituality to sexuality, and while that was okay, she was still unable to handle both. She had sex with whoever she wanted, and it didn't matter to her anymore. I went back home and sat down to evaluate what struck me.

I thought about it that even religions are not against sex. Most care about not doing it outside of marriage because they consider it sacred. Spirituality, more than religiosity, is simply about transcending beyond your physical self and aligning with your spiritual self, your divine. So I said that if I feel entirely at peace with myself and have the values central to sexuality and spirituality, who says practicing sexuality and spirituality is impossible?

As humans, we've all been influenced by society, religious beliefs, our families, or cultural beliefs, whatever it is. Significantly growing up as kids, we had watched our family members or people around us carry out specific actions and express ideas in specific things or practices. Children like to mimic a lot, and it's a primary reason we're who we are today, having values differing slightly or entirely from one another. Some women grew up being told by their parents or guardians that sex was sinful. They told them these lies to prevent them from having sex, but it usually proved abortive because most of these women later grew up to realize these lies and defied them.

But again, all homes are different in their way. Some homes celebrate sex and encourage their children to engage in it with someone special. It all boils down to your attitudes towards things around you, sex inclusive, which your spiritual belief can guide.

How Spirituality Can Influence A Woman

Sexuality and spirituality are very powerful forces, and both can help us understand the complexity and mystery of the world we find ourselves in.

Spirituality can influence a woman in more than one way, but I'd like us to focus on the aspect of sexuality. Spirituality comes with moral values which you're to abide by to live a fulfilling, spiritual life, agreed? When you decide to live a spiritual life, there are many things you might have to set aside to commune with your divine faith. I hope you're getting it? Now sex in its entirety is more than the physical, and these values you now abide by as a result of your sexuality are a part of your sexual experience.

Spirituality can influence a woman who has sex randomly and without a condom. It can influence whether or not to have sex with just anyone, whether or not to use birth control, and even how we handle our relationships. So engaging in sexual activities that contradict the values you abide by will certainly affect your health.

For instance, your spiritual values could be a commitment to one sexual partner, being honest, loyal, etcetera. The moment you step outside that circle and do otherwise, you've created a gap, and negative emotions will set in. You could have feelings of guilt, fear, and self-loathe. This is how spirituality can influence you as a woman.

It is important to understand the values of spirituality and practice them faithfully. Also, note that our faith can change over time, likewise becoming stronger as we grow older.

Sexuality and Spirituality; One Side of a Coin?

I'm about to discuss sexuality and how it affects spirituality, but I need to bring back some definitions to make things easier. In chapter one of this book, I talked about spirituality being "the search for one's inner wealth," seeking "a meaningful connection with something beyond the physical, which causes positive emotions such as peace, contentment, gratitude, and acceptance." Spirituality is about deciding to transcend above our physical self and keying into our spiritual self, our true form that is keen on nothing but positivity. I've talked a lot about spirituality with you and why you need to embrace your spirituality as a black woman to be the best version of yourselves, to allow love to come in, not just to ourselves alone but to others.

Now I'm going to introduce sexuality, which I'm guessing you know pretty much a lot about after my last talk on it. By the way, how's it going with knowing your sexuality, my beautiful black woman? Have you stopped being confused about who you are, and you're like, "you know what? F*ck it. This is who I am, it's something I've always been, or I'm getting into terms with, and as long as it makes me happy, as long as it makes me feel alive, I'm going to keep being me no matter what."

If you've declared such positivity over your life, I am immensely happy for you, and I can't wait to see you move mountains. Also, if you're still on a journey to finding your sexuality, I want you to know that I have gone through such a stage, I've seen and walked a lot of people through this stage, and while it can be daunting and all confusing, it's only worth celebrating that you decided to at least try. So here's to all strong black women searching for their sexuality. I applaud you, I appreciate you and understand your situation, and I want you to know that you're not alone in this. You're never alone, and all you need is time for things to fall in place by themselves. You've got this, black queen!

I defined sexuality as one of the fundamental forces behind people's thoughts, behaviors, and feelings. It encompasses how procreation occurs and talks about one's psychological and sociological beliefs about sex. Sexuality is regulated by various parts of the brain, which shape the body and mind towards seeking pleasure. I want to state that the entirety of sexuality is about sex, sexual orientation, reproduction, gender identity, and pleasure, and we'll be focusing a bit more on sex in this chapter. I hope you've got your pen ready? Let's jump in!

How Have You Been Having Sex?

A lot, and I mean a whole lot, has been said about the word sex. Different views of sex are flying all over the net, with some viewing it as sacred, and I don't mean it religiously. More like in a way that it is special between partners indulging in it. Most religions proclaim sex outside of marriage as sin, while others view sex as natural and a thing to be celebrated. What do I view sex as?

I think sex is sacred, and that's why I'm even talking about the connection between sexuality and spirituality in the first place. Whatever your view of sex is, even the unmentioned ones in this text, is perfectly okay by me as long as you're fine with it. Either way, we still get to learn about sexuality and spirituality.

Despite all that has been said about sex, with more focus on the negative part, it is key to understand that sex is not going anywhere. Oh yes, it is an essential function of humanity. It's a generally known fact that sex has tons of health benefits. Lowering blood pressure, reducing the likelihood of prostate cancer, and improving cardiovascular health are a few benefits. Sex is physical and spiritual, and before you say, "who the hell is this guy talking about sex being spiritual?" Stay with me a while as I explain what I mean.

Remember me saying spirituality is getting in tune with our inner being? However, did you know that sex is a universal force, not just a force but an immense one? You have sex with a partner for the sake of love, or just casual sex that you may think doesn't mean anything. But what if it did?

It's not just about the moans and all the pleasure you feel at that moment. There's a totality in it. As you touch your partner's body, you touch their mind and heart, and more often not, these sexual intercourses leave lasting impressions on your innermost selves. Let me break it down.

If you've had sex, this illustration should be easy to understand.

Have you ever been in a position where after intercourse with your partner, you feel at peace and somewhat joyful, like you're on top of the world? You feel like your spirits are connected, and it's not just about you anymore. You're constantly looking for ways to make your partner happy in several ways. Or maybe not. Maybe none of these happen, and you feel a completely different way. You've not linked your sexuality to your spirituality, and here, my beautiful black queen, is where the link between sexuality and spirituality comes in.

The Link Between Sexuality And Spirituality

Spirituality is about discovering who you truly are — looking into your inner being where there's purity and sexuality is a vital part of it.

During or after spiritual sex, you feel loved and content and, like I said, at peace with your being. A woman who's at peace with herself will willingly contribute to the welfare of others. Most times, people at peace and content with themselves care less about the vain things of life like going after power and fame, material possessions, etc.; all they wish to do is to keep basking in the freedom they've found for themselves while spreading values like love, humility, compassion, and respect.

Woody Harrelson said, "When I was in my twenties and just so sexually prolific, the first time I went to Machu Picchu, this guy, a spiritual teacher, says to me, "When you make love, you must be making love." I thought that was the greatest advice I had ever heard." The link between sexuality and spirituality is the concepts is orgasm, sex, and love. Like what the spiritual teacher said about making love, it's truly important not just to have sex with someone random, but with a partner you're sure is the one for you. A partner you genuinely love and are certain that the feeling is mutual. That way, you're able to make love, and on getting to orgasm, you harness the full potential of your sexual energy.

When I talk about sexuality and spirituality, I do not mean the casual sex that many people in this generation indulge in. Don't get me wrong; I'm not condemning anyone. Whatever you feel is best for you, I'm solidly behind you that you go for it as long as you're not hurting anyone. But I wish to clear your mind that sexuality and spirituality can only be linked when there's love and orgasm, and I don't mean some orgasm you reach through a stranger or someone you don't love, but with someone you don't love.

Having spiritual sex with someone you truly love can positively affect your relationship and cause you both to become more intimate and connected.

Spiritual Women and Sex

I didn't forget we're talking about women, so the focus is on you now. From research, I found out that spirituality has greater consequences among young adults, especially women – than religion. Due to the topic, I went on to study research at a University here in the US and got to interview up to a hundred students, more than half of which were women. I asked them about their thoughts on spirituality, and surprisingly, most of them knew and took their spirituality seriously. The ones who did acknowledge that it helps them experience this sense of fulfillment and somehow connects them emotionally to all of humanity.

"If we want the world to be a better place, let's all get in tune with our spirituality." One of the women had started, and it struck a chord.

As for the males and their responses, the majority of the males didn't see a link between sexuality and spirituality, and genuinely, it's harder for men to see sexuality as spiritual because that's how they're built. A woman can crave intimacy with her partner, and all a man would be thinking of is how to climax and get the urge out of him. He can do this with anyone and not feel attached to his partners, but it's a lot harder for women, hence why it's easier for women to accept that there's a thing as spiritual sex.

Studies show that practicing yoga and other physical activities that promote mental fitness have helped many women who were formally sexually unsatisfied experience a greater level of arousal and orgasms. Spiritual women may also feel comfortable having many sex partners and not see the need to use a condom.

A lingering question might be bugging you at the back of your mind, just like it did years ago. Is it spirituality that makes women want more sex?

Good thing I now have an answer for that.

Scientists have revealed that physical exercises and meditation can set you on a path to bliss, and orgasms help in the effective relief against body pains. Hence, the desire for sex among those connected to the spiritual part of themselves. Having deep conversations about sex with your partner and just talking about ways of improving your sex life can profoundly affect your relationship. So spirituality in itself can spur a woman to want more sex since it connects her to your divine and her partner every time you do.

Using Your Sexuality to Attain Spirituality

As we converse, dear beautiful black woman, we'll be engaging in some practicals, most of which would require you to imagine. Cool, isn't it?

I need you to imagine yourself with your partner and in the mood for sex. They are caressing you and making you feel completely loved and in the spotlight with every touch of theirs. There's so much spark or sexual energy in you, and you feel yourself experiencing pleasure and an emotional connection to your partner. Every detailed touch they give strengthens these feelings, and all you can feel is the unification of your body, mind, and spirit with your partner. Take your imagination up and focus on the period of orgasm, where everything seems timeless, and it's like you've lost yourself in your partner.

Orgasm is got from a French word, 'Orgasmós,' which means 'excitement' and 'swelling.' The French call it 'La petite mort,' which translates to "the little death." Wikipedia says this expression means "the brief loss or weakening of consciousness." During orgasm, a woman loses consciousness for a brief moment and transcends to a state of bliss where she doesn't have to worry about anything.

Now tell me, during your orgasm, did you think about the bills you haven't paid? Or the debtor who's yet to pay?

I don't know about you, but I don't think about my problems. All I can feel is unity with myself, my partner, and the universe. That feeling is what it means to be awakened spiritually. I know these feelings can be short-lived but picture and view them as enlightenments of what being connected to the universe can truly feel like.

When I say using your sexuality to attain your spirituality, I'm talking about viewing sex as something other than a mere physical interaction, like a spiritual practice, like the yoga and meditation exercises you do. If you want to be connected to your partner and feel like one with him, then I'll sexual spirituality is the most effective way.

One time, I had so many bills, all coming after the other, piling up and causing my blood pressure to rise. My cousin was sick, and all I could do was worry about him. My partner came over and saw me in that state. She smiled, and the next thing she did was place her lips on mine. She kissed me and told me that sex helped to reduce stress. I found it funny because I knew that, but up till that moment, I had doubts about it.

As I made love to her, I could feel all the pressure and thoughts evaporating, and I was instantly in nirvana when I experienced orgasm.

Sex can take you to beautiful places you've only imagined. It gives you the feeling that nothing is wrong and happiness rests within your human form and lifetime.

Some women have no personal idea of sex. All they wish to do is satisfy their partners to make the relationship work, no matter what it costs them. You can call them partner pleasers. Haha! It's a term I coined by myself. They're afraid of rocking the boat and would rather see themselves drown in the sea of frustration and dissatisfaction. I wish you to deal with this and get past these terrible feelings. Understand that sex isn't something you need to give others without you benefiting from it. Take time to learn about what you want and what your body desires, and commit to sexual encounters to boost morale and connect you to yourself and your partner.

You automatically reconnect to the divine or universe as you connect to yourself and your partner. When the parties involved intentionally connect to their spirituality, then sex becomes something more than physical activity.

This, my beautiful black woman, is what spiritual sex is about.

Sex As a Physical Activity And Spiritual Practice

You may be wondering what the difference is. Isn't sex just sex? The truth is that sex can be whatever you see it as. I choose to see it as a spiritual practice. It doesn't mean others see it that way, but as a woman on her journey to spirituality, I advise that you navigate your belief into seeing sex as a spiritual practice.

What is the difference?

The difference between physical and spiritual sex lies in whether it is casual or conscious.

An instance would be when you easily vibe to the lyrics of one of the songs of your favorite artist anytime it comes up on the radio. Fine, you know it verbatim, but that's where it ends. You don't make an effort to stream or download the song, but you can openly brag that it's your favorite song. Another instance is when you stream the music, save up to attend live performances by your favorite artist, and stay updated with their lifestyle.

These examples perfectly describe how casual sex and conscious sex are different. You can guess correctly that the first instance is what casual sex is about, while the second is about mindful sex.

In our world today, many people prefer to engage in casual sex because why not? It's less stressful, there are no commitments, and you don't have to feel the headache that comes with giving your all, but in the end, there remains a void that only conscious sex can fill.

Conscious sex provides for intimacy, and when everything is correct, you get to feel complete and at peace, and eventually, casual sex will no longer appeal to you. Who wants to listen to music on the radio when it can stream the song and be comfortable?

A wiki definition of casual sex is any "sexual activity outside a romantic relationship and implies an absence of commitment, emotional attachment, or familiarity between sexual partners." People who engage in casual sex only focus on getting their desires met, either physical or emotional.

Conscious sex, on the other hand, is about creating a connection with your partner to reconnect your body, mind, and spirit to the divine. After sex, it's no longer about you but your connection to someone else and the universe. This spirituality gives sex a whole new meaning.

How To Get In Tune With Your Spirituality Through Sex

To do this, you would need to drop that casual sex and pick up the art of conscious sex. Let's go, black queen!

Be Certain

First things first, ask yourself specific questions. Are you ready to become connected to someone? Will you be comfortable talking about your desires and needs and listening to your partner?

I know how much I've said that sex is more than a physical experience for me, and, to be honest, this repetition is essential. Sex connects you to your partner and is not a sport or something to jump into because you're horny. It'll be better to engage in self-love rather than have casual sex and desire spirituality where you do not have to gamble with someone else's emotions. So my beautiful black woman, be sure that you're ready to have a part of someone in you and a part of you in someone before letting them in.

Also, you do not have to let the propaganda about sex get to you. You do not have to feel ashamed for having sex. It's a beautiful, wonderful experience that should be consensual and free.

Mutual Affection

Sex would be lacking if you or your partner went into it for self-gratification. Spiritual sex should include both partners being intentional and deciding to make the experience worthwhile.

Take away all distractions and communicate with your partner to make sure they're finding the experience pleasurable just as you are. Make sure they're comfortable, and just as you're doing this, they should return the same energy. Sex would be great if we all showed mutual affection to our partners, and we would get in touch with our spirituality that way.

You're Both Divine Manifestations of God

Don't forget spirituality is keying into your inner being and connecting your body, mind, and spirit with the divine. Once you're spiritual, you become a divine manifestation, so I encourage you to view them as such when considering who to choose as a sex partner. Just as you are a divine manifestation of a higher force, so is your partner.

Strive to understand and not judge them. Sex is like a worship of the divine. Your partner with whom you have sex represents the divine, and by connecting your spirit to them, you connect to the divine.

Meditation

As you have sex, it's important not to drift out of the moment. Try as much as you can to focus your attention on your body and observe the sensations you feel.

Consider sex as a meditation. Rather than putting all your effort into achieving orgasm, why not focus on the pleasure you give and receive?

It's essential to experiment with your bodies. Communicate about what turns you on and if you feel your mind drifting away, remember to bring back your focus.

Motive

Before having sex, be sure of your motives and your partner's. If you have different reasons, it won't lead to spirituality. For instance, if one of you wants to have sex for fun while the other wishes for something more, you can make the best bet what's going to happen to the relationship.

I'd love you to understand that you can have casual sex with someone you love and conscious sex with someone you just met. It all boils down to your intention. What do you want?

Do you desire to have a spiritual experience through sex? Then it's best to be intentional about it.

If you're going to have sex for fun, talk it out with your partner. If you're genuinely hoping it'll lead to the start of something great, communicate.

Expectations

Ask yourself how you would like this experience to end. Then ask your partner. Do you both share the exact expectations?

Make sure you still feel the same way you felt initially and do not want to run away after sex. That may just be a sign that you're having casual sex.

Twelve Months Transformation Journal

Finally, we've come to the last segment of your journey, but I'd like to urge you not to feel pressured to start this transformation journal with me until you're ready because it will take commitment and zeal to go through with it every day. Don't forget that it transcends beyond that. Spirituality is a part of living, and this is just a guideline to help you walk that part for as long as you please. I'm sure that it would have become a lifestyle before these fifty-two weeks elapsed.

I've made this journal into a weekly journal to make things easier for you. Each week has seven different activities you're to do every day for us to make significant progress. Don't forget to make the most of this journal. Make it your companion and mentor.

One last thing – have fun!

Week One: Meeting With Your Spirituality

Activity One – It Is Your Journey Alone

Make it a mission today to understand and always remember that this is a journey of self-discovery; hence only you can truly discover yourself.

Choosing to be like someone is okay, but it's essential not to neglect your true capabilities.

Activity Two – Find A Watchword

So your second activity for the week is to find a watchword that you can stick to. It could be a phrase, slogan, or even a quote, anything at all.

Pasting it on your board is a tip to help you remember it faster.

Activity Three – Affirmations

Declare positivity in your life. You're a goal-getter, beautiful, and on a journey to self-discovery and will come out a badass, you know, words like these. Hype yourself always, black queen.

Activity Four – Meditate

Take out about fifteen minutes for yourself and meditate. Chanting or mindfulness can also help calm your mind. Don't forget to do this daily.

Activity Five – Exercise

Your mind alone shouldn't be the only part of you at peace. Let your body feel powerful. Do exercises, yoga, drum, sing, dance even!

Activity Six – Laugh It Out

Laughter, they say, is the best medicine, and I subscribe to that. Don't be so uptight always. If something silly or embarrassing happens, laugh it out. It brings joy.

Activity Seven – Go Over The Activities

I'd love to know what watchword you found.

What were the words you declared about yourself?

How did the meditation go?

I hope you had fun while exercising? If you haven't exercised for a while, you'll need some time to adjust, but you'll be fine.

Laugh!

Week Two: Feeding Your Mind

Activity One – Read A Book

Your guess was right; that was the first thing I would say. Yes, spend at least thirty minutes of your time reading daily.

Activity Two – Listen To A Podcast

Listening to podcasts while exercising, walking, or doing random things will tremendously enrich your mind.

Activity Three – Watch A Documentary

Have you tried Netflix or Amazon Prime documentaries if you find the regular documentary boring? Spiced! Remember, feed your mind.

Activity Four – Question Your Beliefs

You could start by questioning what you were taught in childhood. When you ask questions, you become curious for answers. In finding solutions, you'll be sure to get some new knowledge.

Activity Five – Games

If you're a gamer, I suggest including brain teasers in your collection. I think they're great for developing your brain.

Activity Six – Stop The Comparison

You're only hurting yourself by comparing yourself to others. Experience genuine authenticity and self-love when you stop the comparison.

Activity Seven – Connect With Like-Minded People

If you wish, join a book club, go-to hangout spots, and relax with people who think like you. It's refreshing.

Week Three: Trying Something New

Activity One – Make a list.

 Write out a list of things you'd love to do, learn, places you'd love to visit, and people you'd love to meet. Make a neat list.

Activity Two – Make A Choice

It's time to arrange your list in the order of priority and choose which one to begin with.

Activity Three – Find Out The Obstacles

Determine what the obstacles to achieving these goals would be. Time, money, fear, etc

Activity Four – Draft A Plan

Make a plan on how you can overcome these obstacles. You could save up some money, create time out of your schedule, and be determined. Setting deadlines can help a great deal, but if it would make you feel pressured, I'd instead you don't.

Activity Five – Seek Support

If it would make you feel better to talk to someone about your plan, go for it. Surround yourself with people who would readily support your dreams.

Activity Six-Step Out!

Take that action now. Visit that place, that person. Do what you've always wanted. Step out of your shell.

Activity Seven – Celebrate That Milestone

A round of applause for you on achieving such a feat! You're genuinely a black woman. No matter how little, I truly celebrate you. It would help if you did so too.

Week Four: Achieving Positivity

Activity One – Identify That Negativity

Observe yourself and pick out where you're primarily negative. Now, ask your close friends or spouse about a negative aspect of your life. This part might surprise you.

Activity Two – Find The Root Of Your Negativity

Now that you know the negative aspects of yourself. It's time to deal with the root cause. Take some time to think about what you think could be the cause, then go ahead to tackle it.

Activity Three – Focus On The Good Part

When you're done tackling the negativity, we can now work on achieving positivity. Repeat the same process in activity one and find out yourself. Ask your friends or spouse.

Activity Four – Express Gratitude

Make a list of one thing you're grateful for every day. It enhances awareness of self and things surrounding you.

Activity Five – Laugh And Laugh Again

I will recommend this in many activities for different weeks because I can't stress the importance enough. Even when you don't feel like it, attempt to laugh. It gets easier with time.

Activity Six – Take It Easy

Take it easy on yourself. Try not to let your anger out on yourself when things infuriate or sadden you by self-inflicting damage or harsh words.

Activity Seven – Seek Professional Help

If you don't see progress in your journey to positivity and feel there's a lot more, I urge you to seek professional help as soon as you can. You'd feel much better.

Week Five: Embracing Nature

Activity One – Understand Nature And How It Affects You

I might have to talk about this extensively someday, but you have to do your research for now. Understand how essential nature is to you if you're to find this week interesting.

Activity Two – Narrow The Question To Yourself

When you research, you will find things about the beauty of nature. Now it's time to ask yourself what you love about nature. You don't have to force things; go slowly.

Activity Three – Find Your Nature Spot

It would help a great deal to find a great place in nature where you can meditate or exercise. It doesn't have to be so far away. And no, I'm not giving any suggestions. I'm leaving you to figure this out by yourself, beautiful queen.

Activity Four – Make It A Habit

If you haven't been doing so much in nature, you will have to challenge yourself to develop the habit. Relaxing outside, eating outside, gardening, anything to can think of.

Activity Five – It's The Quality That Matters

It's usually not about how long you spend being in nature but the quality. It wouldn't make sense that you're essential with your mind joggled up with many thoughts. Be in nature and feel at peace.

Activity Six – Sticky Notes

I said sticky notes, and we know what they mean, reminders. If you have a busy schedule, you can place a sticky note on your refrigerator or anywhere you quickly go. Also, your phones can help too.

Activity Seven – Relax

Has it been one hell of a week? It's time to do nothing but relax in nature. Go for an outdoor retreat, step out in the morning, and hang out with a nature buddy. Just relax.

Week Six: Feeding Your Body

Activity One – Always Eat Breakfast

Most people skip breakfast because they're busy or think it helps them lose weight, but you need a breakfast rich in high fiber and low in sugar, fat, and salt for a balanced diet. You can research healthy breakfast ideas and map out a food timetable to follow.

Activity Two – Drink Water

Health experts recommend that you drink a lot of water daily with an average of 8 glasses which should equal 2 liters of water. Never let yourself get dehydrated.

Activity Three – Eat Lots Of Fruits And Veggies

It is recommended that you eat lots of fruits every day. Make it a duty to eat at least five portions of a type of fruit. Also, don't forget to include vegetables in your food.

Activity Four – Eat More Fish

Fish gives protein, a necessary food class, and is needed for a healthy balanced diet. You're also advised to eat oily fish as it contains omega-3 fats, which are suitable for helping to prevent heart disease.

Activity Five – Use Less Salt

Excess salt intake can increase your heart blood pressure, leading to heart disease or even stroke. So as you cook and eat, pls try to make use of less salt.

Activity Six – Reduce Your Saturated Fat And Sugar Intake

Excess saturated fat increases the amount of cholesterol in your blood system, which can also cause heart disease. Reduced saturated fat intake means cutting down on foods like butter, hard cheese, cakes, etc.

Also, note today that excess sugar can increase your risk of tooth decay and obesity.

Activity Seven – Exercise

Lastly, I'd love for you to begin exercising daily for this week. No matter how fit you think you are, exercising, just like eating healthy foods, can help reduce the risk of obesity and other diseases, especially heart diseases.

Week Seven: Practicing Gratitude

Activity One – Understand Why You Should Practice Gratitude

I do not wish to impose my beliefs on you, so it's only proper that I enlighten you on why you should practice gratitude.

Gratitude significantly boosts happiness, helps you feel more positive emotions, and improves your relationship with others, among a host of other benefits. So I'll implore you to do your research and decide to embark on this journey to practice gratitude or not.

Activity Two – Have A Journal

I expect that by now, you have a journal you're working with for your spirituality. Another separate journal, however, is also a good idea in your journey to expressing gratitude.

Activity Three – Be Specific About What You're Grateful For

I'd like you not just to express gratitude but to be particular about your expression. If you're thankful for something, write it down. For example: "I'm thankful that I am in this situation today," or "I am thankful that I made a lot of progress in my work today."

Activity Four – Go Into Detail

Saying something isn't usually enough. To practice gratitude, you should explain what you are grateful for and why you are. You don't feel like it's an obligation to express gratitude.

Activity Five – Don't Ignore The Negative.

When your life is going so well, don't forget the times when things were rough because it is in that forgetfulness that pride sets in. Remembering how you came to a certain level would help you express gratitude.

Activity Six – Use Reminders

At times you may tend to forget about what you've achieved or what someone has done for you and not express gratitude when you should. Using visual reminders and asking yourself questions like "What has this person given to me?" "Have I achieved a goal I should be grateful for?" etc., would help a great deal.

Activity Seven – Express Gratitude Outwardly

Once you've been grateful inwardly, like expressing gratitude in your journal and all of that, you're ready for the outside world. Use words like "Thank you," "I appreciate what you've done for me," etc., to build stronger relationships with people.

Week Eight: Voicing Out Affirmations

This week will be a bit different from the rest because the entire week will be about affirmations on various subjects. I'll list out three but feel free to add as much as you desire!

Activity One – Affirmations For Health

"I am grateful for my body."

"Whatever I feel in my body, I will tend to it with utmost care and precision, never judging or being hard on my body."

"I am open to new ways of living a healthy lifestyle."

Activity Two – Affirmations For Love

"I let go of every negativity that came with my past love, and I am willing to receive a new love."

"I am ready to stay committed to nurturing the heart."

"I deserve all the love I'm being showered because I return just as much."

Activity Three – Affirmations For Self-Esteem

"I deserve to get everything I desire."

"I will soar above the sky and achieve all my goals."

"I am a brilliant woman and the most beautiful."

Activity Four – Affirmations For Self-Love

"I choose not to give in to stress and self-harm."

"Whenever I feel stressed, I'll always remember to pause and take a deep breath."

"No one is perfect. I acknowledge my mistake and admit my flaws. However, I'm not letting it get to me. I will try again."

Activity Five – Affirmations For Peace And Harmony

"I've begun my spiritual journey and will strive to attain inner peace."

"I have a good relationship with my friends and family. I love them, and they love me."

"Everything is in perfect control."

Activity Six – Affirmations For Joy And Happiness

"Everything right now is working for my good."

"I am a happy woman."

"I am full of joy and happiness; therefore, I will live longer."

Activity Seven – Affirmations For Anxiety

"Everything seems as though it's tumbling, but I choose to be calm."
"Things eventually turn out to be okay in the end. I have to take a deep breath."

"I'm overthinking right now. I should stop it."

Week Nine: Finding Peace Amidst Chaos

Activity One - Get Occupied

It doesn't necessarily mean working or doing something strenuous, watching your favorite tv shows, drawing, dancing, engaging in karaoke, hanging out, etc. Any fun thing you love to do to distract you.

Activity Two – Stop Consuming Negativity

Some people tend to self-destruct when they're faced with challenges. If social media is the primary source of negativity in your life, it's better to take a break. Walk away from anything that doubles your sadness.

Activity Three – Get Rid Of The Stress

If you're feeling stressed, you could take a walk, jog, go on a vacation, exercise, or any other idea you have of ridding of stress.

Activity Four – Refine Your Brain With Positive Affirmation

Remember last week; I gave some affirmations about peace and anxiety. Claims of peace should help you control your emotions.

Activity Five – Stop Doubting

If you approach a situation with doubt in your mind, there's a high chance that you aren't going to make the best of it. So whatever you're going through, you have to approach it with courage and hope that things will fall into place.

Activity Six – Focus On Your Purpose

Things are tough right now, but you have a goal to achieve and a purpose of fulfilling. It wouldn't be right for you to give up. Take a break, find calm in that raging storm but don't give up.

Activity Seven – Seek Help

It could be your problem is beyond all of these solutions, but this last one should do the trick. Talk to someone, a friend, family, or professional. Let them know what you're going through and seek advice from them.

Week Ten: Read A Book

Activity One – Decide

Before buying your book, you have to skim through the contents and decide which book you will read for the entire week. Then make that purchase.

Activity Two – Reason For Choice

What made you decide to get that particular book? Can you write what intrigues you most about the text in your journal? I'd also love to hear it if you can.

Activity Three – Jot Down As You Read

Jotting down can help you remember points you've learned from the book. Also, jotting down new words would help expand your vocabulary and keep you abreast with ideologies.

Activity Four – Relax Your Mind

Don't feel pressured to read if you don't feel like it. Make sure you're calm and begin reading if you're to get value from the book you're reading effectively.

Activity Five: Put Into Practice What You've Learnt.

Remember the words you jotted down? It's time to reread them. Try to use those new words in your everyday conversations. Also, the moral lessons you've learned should be put into practice.

Activity Six – Finding A Reading Partner

At times you may feel alone when you start reading a book. Finding someone who finds interest in reading will help a great deal in boosting your interests. Your partner can cheer you up when the need arises and recommend great books for you.

Activity Seven – Join A Book Club

Book clubs are great places to go to broaden your knowledge of books and spike up your interests.

Week Eleven: Adopting The Virtue Of Forgiveness

Activity One – Accept That Everyone Makes Mistakes.

This is one of the first steps taken to forgiveness. Realizing that no one is above mistakes makes you understand that you can make mistakes too and will want to be forgiven. This should make forgiveness relatively easy for you.

Activity Two – Mistakes Are A Part Of Life

No matter how we try to shy away from the truth, the reality will always be that mistakes are s part of life and will frame whatever we might become in the future, depending on how we take it.

Activity Three – Don't hold Grudges.

Have you been offended by anyone? No matter who that person may be, let them know that they have crossed a line they shouldn't have. Please don't keep it to yourself.

Activity Four – Forgive Others

The gravity of an offense could make this very hard to do. But it'll be the best decision you will ever make. The freedom that comes with forgiveness is limitless.

Activity Five – Forgive Yourself.

You probably have done something that you weren't proud of in the distant past and recent past. You've got to let go of yourself too. It's not the end of the world.

Activity Six – Make Amends

If you're not making progress from your mistakes, you're making a more significant mistake, and that's not the woman you are. Make amends and grow stronger every day.

Activity Seven – Affirmation

I have mistakes too, and as I forgive myself, I will also ignore the people around me who have offended me. That's how I want to live my life.

Week Twelve: Adopting the Virtue of Prudence

Activity One – Understanding Prudence

Prudence is the virtue of being careful about the choices you make. Stopping to think about your next move and not taking unnecessary risks. It is a virtue of careful thinking for better decision-making.

Activity Two - Understanding The Need To Be Prudent

Why should you be prudent? The life you see can happen to anyone at any time. You wouldn't want to overlook that because one careless decision can cost you more than you can even imagine.

Activity Three – Counsel Yourself

Taking any crucial decision in your life requires you to brainstorm extensively. Don't ever rush to make decisions you might regret later. Making decisions on impulse could be fatal.

Activity Four – Seek Counsel From Others

You're not alone in the world. If you feel that you're at crossroads and don't know what to do, seek help from those you think are capable of helping you.

Activity Five – Learn From Your Past

You have made mistakes in the past and gained knowledge in the process. Use that knowledge when the need arises so that you don't make the same mistake twice.

Activity Six – Weighing Your Risks and Rewards.

To make decisions carefully, weighing your risks and rewards can be a handy tool. Ask yourself, this risk I am about to take, is it worth the reward? The answer to that question can shape your thought process and enable you to make good decisions.

Activity Seven – You Are Responsible For The Consequences Of Your Actions

Whenever you want to make a decision, always remember that you will be held liable for whatever action you take after you have made your decision.

Week Thirteen – Adopting The Virtue Of Temperance

Activity One - Understanding The Virtue Of Temperance

This, in simpler terms, is a virtue of restraint, and it is based on particularly whatever an individual seeks to refrain from doing. It could be alcoholism, extravagant spending, or whatever vice an individual deems not worthy of doing.

Activity Two – Identifying Toxic Traits

Identifying those things you want to refrain from is a start of a good foot to abstaining from them. If you don't know what you want, you can hardly achieve anything.

Activity Three - Acknowledging Your Toxic Traits

This may look like the previous subtopic, but a thin line differentiates them. It's not healthy to deceive yourself. When you know that you have a toxic trait, say, alcoholism, you shouldn't lie to yourself about it. By acknowledging your condition, you make it easy to make efforts to refrain.

Activity Four – Have Them Written Down

This is a very underrated activity. Get a journal just like this, one; of the things you wish to refrain from; go through them at the start of your day to remind yourself and see how well you fared at the end of the day.

Activity Five – Monitor Your Progress

From time to time, look back at how you've been faring. How have things changed? How often did you go clubbing and get wasted? When was the last time you rolled a joint? Question yourself about the journey.

Activity Six – Celebrate Your Progress

Commend yourself for a job well done with each step you take up the ladder to Temperance. This doesn't mean you should throw a party or something. It is something that happens from within. Even a smile of satisfaction would do.

Activity Seven – Don't Be So Hard on Yourself.

The journey would not be a linear one. One after the other. No-no-no. You'll fall back sometimes, but you always have to stay calm and not be hard on yourself. You're human.

Week Fourteen – Adopting The Virtue Of Justice

Activity One – Understanding The Virtue of Justice

In human relations, justice means giving each person what they deserve. Not treating everyone the same, but treating them accordingly. It would help if you understood that equality is not justice.

Activity Two – Applying Justice To Your Self Improvement

This virtue may not only pertain to your relationship with humans. You can apply justice to your personal life. This means things that you do that are important to you. It could be education, a craft, your work, workouts, and many others.

Activity Three – Knowing How To Do Justice To Your Everyday Living.

The previous chapter spoke about justice being applied to other spheres of life. Here is a simple formula to help you streamline your activities so that you'd be doing justice to them; Focus your attention on the things you know will benefit you in the long run. They are deserving of your attention, and that's what justice entails.

Activity Four – Knowing How To Do Justice To People

This should be simple. Go all out for the people that do the same for you. Make time for the people that do the same for you. There's no time trying to impress who wouldn't even care. Show love to those that are deserving of it.

Activity Five – Studying How You Relate With People

Have you closely watched how you relate with people wherever you go? Church, School, Workplace? What are the patterns that you have noticed? Could you take note of them?

Activity Six – Study The Patterns

The patterns that you have noticed, you have to study them to decipher the loopholes. Are you treating people based on their race, gender, financial status, or political power? That would be unfair to them. On the other hand, are you giving too much attention to those who care about you and neglecting those who do? That'll be unfair to yourself.

Activity Seven – Work On Improvement

What's a study without usage? You know what ought to be and ought not. So make use of that knowledge from studying the patterns to improve yourself.

Week Fifteen – Adopting The Virtue Of Fortitude

Activity One – Understanding The Virtue of Fortitude

One of the visible traits of a black woman is Fortitude. It means that one manages to be solid or courageous even amid adversity and pain.

Activity Two – Understanding That Life Is Full Of Challenges

Even for the children born into wealthy homes, life would still be full of challenges. No man has lived an entirely peaceful life till he died. If you don't understand that, you should now.

Activity Three – Understanding The Need To Have Fortitude

Some may be asking, why do I need to show strength while passing through adversity? If you're one of those, don't forget to ask yourself who'd be willing to associate with a weak person. Whether you like it or not, a courageous person would get help before the one who is timid and weak.

Activity Four – You Can't Be 100% Ready

There are some setbacks you don't see coming, and they can be very devastating when they hit you. That's one thing you have to understand as you journey through life so that you don't wear yourself out with standards that are impossible to attain.

Activity Five – It's Okay To Stay Down For A While

It would be a different situation entirely if you saw it coming. But if you didn't, you may have to chill for a bit. Not forever, though. Just a little break enough to get you back in some shape.

Activity Six – Confide In People

It could be a partner, parent, or friend. It's possible to draw strength from them while maintaining yours. Never be too shy to talk if you can't take it all in. You don't want to go crazy, do you?

Activity Seven – Celebrate Your Wins

Yes! I repeat this. When you're finally able to get through that situation, give yourself some credit. It boosts your morale and assures you that you can do it through the next challenge.

Week Sixteen – Adopting The Virtues Of Goodness And Compassion

Activity One – Understanding The Virtues Of Goodness and Compassion

Having goodness and compassion means being generous and kind to people around you. With your words and with your actions without expecting anything in return.

Activity Two – Understand Why You Should Be Good To People

Doing an act of kindness from a genuine heart makes you happy and fulfilled. That's enough reason to be good to people. Imagine what joy you'd feel when you see the smile on the face of an older woman who you just gave alms. That alone can make your day!

Activity Three – Saying Kind Words

The tongue can cut like a knife if misused. You don't know what that person might be going through. Always be kind with your words. You might be saving a life.

Activity Four – Kind Deeds

You can take out a day or two in the week to carry out acts of kindness. It could be to those you know or not. It doesn't have to cost much—the thought counts.

Activity Five – Acts Of Services

In your workplace, around where you live, in your school, anywhere you find yourself, don't be hesitant to act out acts of service. It could be cleaning the neighborhood or running errands for a coworker.

Activity Six – Be Kind With Your Time

Though it may look immaterial, time is an essential aspect of human life, and being kind with your time will mean a lot to those who'd value it.

Activity Seven – Be Kind To Yourself

While you're being kind to other people, you've got to be kind to yourself. Take yourself out on treats, constantly remind yourself how special you are, and don't let anyone look down on you.

Week Seventeen – Adopting the Virtue of Practical Wisdom

Activity One – Understanding The Virtue of Practical Wisdom

Practical wisdom means knowing how to balance conflicting principles. This kind of wisdom acknowledges that uncertain risk cannot be avoided but guides us in becoming wiser about how we manage it.

Activity Two – Understanding The Need For Practical Wisdom

This virtue helps you balance your risk and take decisions that wouldn't cost much if anything goes south. It is a handy tool when you're at crossroads.

Activity Three – Acknowledge The Need For Practical Wisdom

The need for something creates a longing to get it by all means possible. Everyone needs to know what practical wisdom is, and you'd not be doing yourself a favor by lying to yourself that you don't need it.

Activity Four – Read Books

Books are a very reliable source of knowledge, but you have to make sure you're reading the right ones. Dedicate a month to complete a book, jot down what you've learned, and visit them regularly.

Activity Five – Seek Advice From Experienced People

There's no harm in going to others to seek advice. It's better than going headlong into what you know nothing about and failing.

Activity Six – Learn From Experience

Your past is a teacher. Please take advantage of everything it has to teach you because you paid heavily for it with the consequences of any mistake you made back then.

Activity Seven: Put What You've Learnt Into Practice.

Don't just sit there learning. Why would it be called Practical Wisdom when you're not going to act? The real benefit of your knowledge is in its application. Never forget that.

Week Eighteen – Adopting The Virtue of Humility

Activity One – Understanding The Virtue Of Humility

Humility is the virtue of being humble and putting another person's interest over yours. But don't be quick to equate this to having low self-esteem. That's far from it.

Activity Two – Understanding The Need To Be Humble

Humility is an attractive virtue, and it creates a very enabling environment for people around you. No one wants to be around a cocky person who would make people feel less of themselves. I will be highlighting a few ways to practice humility across the remaining activities.

Activity Three – Listening To Others.

Others would see what you may be doing wrong before you do. Always give listening ears to what others have to say to you. It allows you to learn more about yourself.

Activity Four – Cultivate The Act Of Gratitude

Be grateful for what you have and what you've achieved. I get it. You may have had a lot to do with your success, but don't ever forget that some force beyond the physical has enabled you to achieve that which others failed at.

Activity Five – Ask For Help When You Need It

Don't die in silence. If you need help, reach out to others to help you through that difficult phase. You're not alone in this world, and in one way or the other, the impact of others must be felt in your life.

Activity Six – Don't Be Too Quick To Judge.

This activity applies to both other people and yourself. Why judge? You may have no idea what the person you're judging is going through. Be humble enough to accept the person while helping the person improve.

Activity Seven: Appreciate The Effort Of Others.

No matter how insignificant it may seem, You must appreciate the efforts of others because you may not be aware of what it took for that person to make such an effort.

Week Nineteen – Adopting The Virtue Of Honesty

Activity One – Understanding The Virtue Of Honesty

Honesty is the virtue of being truthful. To both yourself and others. Saying a thing as it is and not painting it to be something else.

Activity Two – Understanding The Need For Honesty.

You must understand that being honest makes you a more reliable and trustworthy person. It also creates a safe space around you for others to seek opinions.

Activity Three – Staying True To Yourself

Stop trying to be something you're not. It rubs you off your originality, and the world loses your peculiarity because you've become another person.

Activity Four: You Don't Need To Be Brutally Honest.

When telling someone the truth, how you say it to the person is as crucial as the truth itself. You have to say to them as lovingly as possible. Make sure the person doesn't get hurt in the process.

Activity Five – Being Transparent In Your Dealings

Nobody likes a cunning person. If you're not honest in your way of life, no one would want anything to do with you and will be hesitant to offer help when you need it.

Activity Six – Company of Like Minds.

While you strive to be honest, surround yourself with real people. In such a formative period of your life, any form of negativity would dissuade you.

Activity Seven – Embrace Being Honest

Some people are scared of being honest because of what others may have to say. But that shouldn't bother you. You're fighting for the purity of your conscience, and what other people say should matter as long as you're doing the right thing.

Week Twenty – Adopting The Virtue Of Love
Activity One – Understanding The Virtue Of Love

Love is a deep feeling of affection towards a person or yourself. It encompasses some of what we've discussed previously, so this is probably like a recap of the discussion so far.

Activity Two – Forgiveness

You must be willing to forgive those you love and accept yourself more. You have to forgive yourself as well.

Activity Three – Honesty

When you love a person, you seek the overall improvement of such a person, and being honest will help you achieve that.

Activity Four – Goodness/Compassion

When you are in a position to help, it becomes straightforward to help such a person out in times of their need or even randomly.

Activity Five – Patience

Loving a person requires a lot of patience, tolerance, and overlooking a lot of things that are supposed to get you riled up.

Activity Six – Commitment

Commitment is the virtue of being dedicated to a particular cause. Loving a person requires you to be committed to that person's growth and welfare.

Activity Seven – Respect

In this context, we'd be referring to having regard for the feeling of others. You must understand that not everyone would be comfortable with everything you love doing. Recognizing this and acting goes a long way in telling how much you love a person.

Week Twenty-One: Spirituality and Humanitarianism

This week is about learning intensively, so in addition to all I'll be saying throughout the week, I urge you to do extensive research on the following concepts I will briefly talk about.

One week will be majorly theory, while the subsequent week will be practical. I've made it that way so that you find your weeks completely fun, educational, and practicable.

Activity One – Understanding The Concept of Humanitarianism

Although the word isn't so common in everyday usage, I believe you must have heard of it. Today's activity is that you research the meaning of Humanitarianism. I'll give a brief definition, and you can check out others. Wikipedia defines Humanitarianism to be an active belief in the value of human life and the practice of humane treatment and provision of assistance to humans to reduce their suffering. Now, you can pick it up from there.

Activity Two – Relating Humanitarianism To Spirituality

Spirituality is about your connection to your true self, and it extends outwardly and helps you connect with others on a whole new level. When you've attained spirituality, the virtue of benevolence to humans wouldn't be so hard. Find time to get a note on how being a humanitarian can boost your spirituality and vice versa.

Activity Three - Concept Of Tribalism

Ordinarily, the concept of tribalism meant the advocacy for tribes and their lifestyles. But it's now associated with the negative part, which defines it as hostilities towards particular tribes by other groups. Research more on tribalism and instances where it has caused grave damage to people.

Activity Four – Humanitarianism Fights Against Tribalism

Based on the above concept of tribalism to be either advocacy for tribes or hostilities against tribes, Humanitarianism seeks to bring peace amongst various warring tribes and encourage harmony between all tribes. Learn about how Humanitarianism has affected the negative aspects of tribalism in today's world.

Activity Five – Concept Of Slavery

We'll learn about the history of slavery, and I'm keen on seeing you make the best out of this topic. I'll set aside an entire week for activities in which you'll learn about the history and power of black people. But for today's action, I only desire you to learn about the general history of slavery in the world.

Activity Six – Humanitarianism Fights Against Slavery

Slavery might sound archaic because that's how it seems, but did you ever think about the narrative that, although repressed, it still exists and is even revolutionized? That's by the way, though. Before we conclude the week's activities tomorrow, write out ten humanitarians who fought against slavery and try to learn about them.

Activity Seven – Humanitarianism Fights Against Discrimination

Oh, how much I love this part because it would lead us to the practical aspect of this topic for week twenty-one. For today, learn extensively about discrimination, ways people discriminate, and how we can reduce discrimination in our society.

Week Twenty-Two: Practicing Humanitarianism

Activity One – Reach Out

You don't have to fret about the tasks for this week as they'll be straightforward.

Please take notice of a person or persons who always seem left out in your place of work or school and talk to them. Just interact.

Activity Two – Visitations

Find time in your schedule to visit someone in the hospital who is probably, sick, recovering, or nursing. You can also opt to see an older adult who's usually alone.

Activity Three – Invitations

If you're not comfortable with visiting people or do not have the time but prefer accepting visits in your home, you could host a meal and invite a homeless person or less privileged to eat with you.

Activity Four – Donations

You could donate domestic equipment, your blood, toiletry supplies, toys, food boxes, etc. Also, go for other ideas about local donations that come to your mind.

Activity Five – Writing

Publishing articles on Humanitarianism that help enlighten people about the concept and promote it amongst them is a great way. Writing and simply sharing on social media is also a great idea.

Activity Six – Babysitting

Offering to babysit a child whose parents are extremely busy is also a way of showing Love to humans. You can also watch over teenagers and give them good advice.

Activity Seven – Campaign

You can hold a campaign to promote Humanitarianism and broaden people's knowledge on why we should show compassion to ourselves and aim to be better persons.

Week Twenty-Three: Signs To Look For In Spiritual Persons

You might need to talk to certain persons or make friends with people who would help and encourage you on your spiritual journey. The following are ways to recognize a spiritual person.

Activity One – Recognition Of Self

If there's anyone you have in mind to be your mentor or spiritual friend, you have to be able to know if they recognize themselves in others. Do they see themselves as one with all beings, things, and creatures and therefore trail the path of Love and compassion towards all beings? If you see yourself as one with someone, would you want to hurt yourself?

Activity Two – Sincerity And Humility

I want to share this quote by Nisargadatta with you. I found it captivating, so here; "When I look within and see that I am nothing, that's wisdom. When I look out and see that I am everything, that's Love. Between these two, my life turns."

Spiritual people know who they are in this world and understand the need to remain humble and sincere to themselves.

Activity Three – True Lovers

Observe a spiritual person and notice how they love. There are no strings attached, and they love freely. They're the embodiment of Love and radiate it in its glory. A spiritual person would not wait for you to show Love to them before they reciprocate. Neither would they stop if you don't return. They are children of Love.

Activity Four – Trust

Spiritual Persons do not worry unnecessarily about what tomorrow holds but rather believe and hope that things will fall in place. They allow life to lead the way.

Activity Five – Search For Their Forgiving Spirit

Spiritual Persons do not expect humans to be perfect and therefore are more than willing to forgive them when they err or mistreat them. This virtue is rare as most people harbor hate in them, so you'll be lucky to find someone with a forgiving spirit.

Activity Six – Generous Hearts

At some point, you may need a favor from your spiritual friend, and one of the ways you can know that they're in tune with their spirituality is in their generosity of heart, giving without asking back.

Activity Seven – Quietness And Solitude

All spiritual persons love to meditate, so this should be easy to spot. I can imagine how happy you would be when you find someone who loves quietness just as you do!

Week Twenty-Four: Spirituality and Environmentalism

Activity One – Understanding The Concept Of Environmentalism

This week is going to be just like week twenty. I hope you remember how it went and all you practiced concerning Humanitarianism. Environmentalism is the concern and actions expressed by people to protect the environment. We'll be doing a lot of theory and practice this week. So today, research on the meaning and history of environmentalism.

Activity Two – Relating Environmentalism To Spirituality

Today will be about understanding the link spirituality has with environmentalism. The knowledge that spirituality has to do with finding our true selves and being in tune with nature is enough for you to begin linking these two concepts together.

Activity Three – Reflection On Our Actions

I'll ask three questions, and you let me fill your journal with seven more reflection questions.

"How do you view the environment around you?"

"Have you supported environmental pollution by your actions, inactions, or words?"

"How do you dispose of your dirt?"

Activity Four – Global Warming

You can write out the definition of global warming, the causes, and the effects. I'll give three examples of global warming:

Shifts in the blooming of flowers.

Continuous decrease in the extent of ice and snow.

Dirtier air.

Activity Five – Steps To Environmentalism

With the assumption that you've studied environmentalism, global warming, and other pollution, the next three days from today will be on the commitment to keeping your environment clean.

For today, conserve water.

Activity Six – Practice The 3Rs

The 3Rs, which I'd like to call Reduce, Reuse, and Recycle, are ways to make your environment better. Reduce the inessential things you buy. Make sure to reuse items that can be reused rather than throwing them away, and lastly, Recycle.

Activity Seven – Conserve Electricity

Research on ways to conserve electricity. Start today with switching off the lights when not in use.

Week Twenty-Five: Practicing Environmental Care

Activity One – Plant a tree today.

Activity Two – Conserve Water

Fix a leaking pipe.

Collect water from the rain and water your lawn with it another day.

Don't leave the tap running while brushing your teeth.

Activity Three – Go environmentally friendly with a Rooftop Solar Photovoltaic (PV). It's affordable.

Activity Four – Change all your bulbs to LED light bulbs today. They last longer and use less power.

Activity Five – Stop wasting food intentionally and unintentionally. Try as much as possible to cook or buy what you can finish.

Activity Six – Use fewer products made of fossil fuels.

Activity Seven – Take a stroll to the nearest grocery store nearby and buy locally grown products. They're completely healthy, plus you're supporting local farms and dairies.

Week Twenty-Six: Spirituality and Mental Health

Activity One – Understanding You're More Important

The most important person in your life is you—work towards truly understanding this and see how much you'd love yourself.

Activity Two – Speak Up

If you're still bothered about something after twenty-four hours, speak up within forty-eight hours.

Activity Three – Stop The Addiction

You could be excessively doing consciously or unconsciously in an attempt to numb pain. But don't you think it's better to speak out or talk to someone about how you truly feel than to do things that would harm you?

Activity Four: Don't Apologize For What You Feel.

Often, you might feel a specific way about something or someone and end up apologizing because you expressed it. If you say it entirely civilized, you do not have to apologize.

It's okay to be sad, happy, terrified, anxious, or any other emotion. You shouldn't apologize for how you feel. Try to build your self-esteem with this and exercise self-control towards your feelings.

Activity Five – You Are Responsible For Yourself

Forget that you have a husband, wife, children, or friend. Do you care for yourself as much as you do for them? Do you take out time for yourself? Giving yourself time gives you peace and helps you connect more with your family and friends.

Activity Six – Go Through Your Pain

Rather than walking away or trying to numb your pain, you should go through it. That way, you're able to overcome it and become stronger.

Activity Seven – Seek Help

When you look at it, asking for help is one of the best steps to success. Rather than doing it all on your own, why not talk to someone to help you with it, help you overcome that feeling? To your greatest surprise, some people want to help.

Week Twenty-Seven: Fixing Your Mental Health

Activity One – Write out ten Affirmations on self-love.

Activity Two – Talk to someone about what they did to offend or hurt you.

Activity Three – Go a day without something you're addicted to. Celebrate that feat and try reducing the addiction.

Activity Four – Meditate today. Write out ten valuable things about yourself.

Activity Five – Do something that involves going through your pain and not walking away from it.

Activity Six – Treat yourself to a nice meal.

Activity Seven – Talk to a friend, family member, or a professional about your feelings.

Week Twenty-Eight: Practicing Self-awareness

Activity One: Meditate on your thoughts daily.

Activity Two: Listen to what others have to say about you.

Activity Three: Travel to places and watch your reactions to these places.

Activity Four: Learn a new skill that would enable you to think and act originally.

Activity Five: Observe what you blurt out when stressed or angry and become more aware of yourself.

Activity Six: Do a quick reflection and write five values you hold in high esteem.

Activity Seven: Try writing fiction or reading a fictional story and observe how you think about certain things.

Week Twenty-Nine: Defining Your Happiness

Activity One – Loving Yourself

When you love and cherish yourself, which spirituality teaches you to, it would be hard to be shaken by what others say or do to you?

Activity Two – Helping Others

Carry out a kind action today.

Activity Three – Acceptance

Look at yourself in the mirror and notice how beautiful you are. Learn to accept all your flaws.

Activity Four – Transcending Materialism

Ask yourself questions about how materialistic you are.

Determine today not to place your happiness on material things.

Activity Five – Celebrate

Write out ten things you achieved the previous week and think of a way to celebrate your success.

Activity Six – Do What You Love

List five things you love doing every time. Make sure to do them every day if possible and keep track of this.

Activity Seven – Make Good Friends

If your friends aren't making you happy, it's time to surround yourself with better people.

Week Thirty: Generosity week!

Activity One – Gifts

Buy someone a dress.

Write someone a handwritten note.

Pay for a stranger's coffee.

Please include some more, my beautiful black woman.

Activity Two – Learning Kind Words

"You always excel at what you do!"

"You are so brave!"

"You are a beautiful human, and I don't mean only on the external. You have a big heart."

Activity Three – Visit A Retirement Home

Go with gifts, of course, and interact with the elderly. Listen to them talk about their experiences, and be sure to get a few life tips from them. You can even ask someone to guide you on your path to spirituality.

Activity Four – Alternatives To Money

If you want to give someone something as an act of kindness this week but do not have the money for it. Here are three alternatives, and of course, you could add yours.

Donate blood to a hospital.

Volunteer your time to the development of your community.

Donate extra belongings. It could be clothes, toys, or pieces of equipment you no longer need.

Activity Five – Compliments

Today is for compliments. Get your journal out and decide to compliment ten strangers today. Please fill up your diary with your choice of compliments and the replies from each of them. This activity should be fun.

Activity Six – Determine To Be Patient

Here's another practice for you. Write out the number of times you got angry over something this week. You don't have to stress over remembering everything. Just the few you remember are okay. Now take up the challenge not to flare up over a trivial issue. Best of luck, brave woman!

Activity Seven: Have some rest.

You've done so much this week, giving, and giving, and I'm proud of you for your progress. You deserve all the rest you can get, but don't forget that each activity is a continuous process. You're not to stop just because the week runs out and another begins with new activities.

Overall, have some fun today and laugh more.

Week Thirty-One: Voicing Out Affirmations 2

It's another special week where we'll be voicing out affirmations. I'll list out three affirmations as usual, and you can add as much as you wish.

Activity One – Affirmations For Leaders

"I am a role model to people, an inspiration."

"I know I can and will make a positive change."

"People will remember me for good."

Activity Two – Affirmations For Black Women

"I love how dark my skin is."

"I know how unique my hair texture is. That's why I'm in love with it."

"I will enact the change I desire."

Activity Three – Affirmations For Working Moms

"My children love and see me as a great parent."

"I make a difference in my family."

"I am supportive and a powerhouse."

Activity Four – Affirmations For Confidence

"I can do difficult tasks."

"I am bright and articulate."

"I believe I can do this."

Activity Five – Affirmations For Honoring Your Achievements

"I am proud of all I've achieved."

"My friends and family will be so proud of me."

"I am a winner, a conqueror."

Activity Six – Affirmations For a Healthy Mindset

"I believe in my abilities."

"I feel safe, happy, and content."

"I am in control of my reaction to others."

Activity Seven – Affirmations For Relationships

"I love my partner."

"I do not envy my partner's success but wish to see them grow."

"I do not have doubts about my partner's fidelity."

Week Thirty-Two: Growing Your Business

Activity One – Meditation

Meditation is a required method of growing your business. Dedicating time to yourself for meditation helps you become aware of yourself and your purpose. Meditation opens your mind to new ideas for your business.

Activity Two – Humility

Nobody likes a person who is proud and boastful. Understand that you're just one in the world and need people to fulfill your existence. So when things are going great for you, don't let it get into your head.

Activity Three – Be Gracious

In all you do, radiate light wherever you are. As you carry out your duties in your business place, do them graciously. Strive to stand out amongst your peers and competitors.

Activity Four – Say Sorry When You Should

If you wrong your customers or fellow humans, apologize instantly and suppress the urge to make up excuses.

Activity Five – Practice Forgiveness

When someone offends you, it's ideal that you let them know and forgive them instantly, whether they apologize. Forgiving people help your mind to stay healthy and encourages your growth.

Activity Six – Stop Limiting Your Thoughts

Deliberately or subconsciously limiting your thoughts and letting doubts is a road to failure. Allow your mind to express its creativity.

Activity Seven – Be Positive

Treat people kindly always, no matter how they may be. When you treat all kinds of people nicely, it makes them feel like you believe in them, possibly that they can be good.

Week Thirty-Three: Spirituality and Career Development

Activity One – Express Positivity

When your co-workers are feeling down due to things happening in your workplace, it's your duty as a spiritual person to offer them comfort and hope that things will get better.

Activity Two – Take Some Time Out

If you're feeling too tired from working continuously, it's okay to take a break. Remember always to meditate.

Activity Three – Connect With Your Co-workers

Being a spiritual person is about connecting with your true self and others, and a great place to connect with people is at your workplace. Bake pie and share with your co-workers, ask them how their day is going, etc.

Activity Four – Share Ideas With Your Boss

It wouldn't be nice if you have a great idea but choose to keep it to yourself. Think of ideas that would boost the company's values and success.

Activity Five – Use Words Carefully

When angry, take a breath before speaking. When stressed, breathe in and out. With any negative emotion you feel within you, always take a breath to think of what to say. Words can scar people for life, so you might want to choose your words more carefully.

Activity Six – Reflection

Take time to reflect on your progress since you started working for the company. Think of things you could do to be rewarded with a promotion. Also, congratulate yourself on your progress so far.

Activity Seven – Host A Party

In the spirit of connecting with your co-workers, hosting a party is a great idea to get together and relax after work.

Week Thirty-Four: Living Healthy Lifestyles

Activity One – Drink More Water

Activity Two – Eat Fruits And Vegetables

Whenever you're at the grocery store, always get fruits to eat after your meal.

Activity Three – Avoid Harboring Negativity

Stop doubting your potential. Stop harboring hate and all other negative emotions. Let go of the negativity in your life.

Activity Four – Get Enough Sleep

If you've not been getting enough sleep, you're not living healthily. Sleep for at least eight hours today and every other day.

Activity Five – Walk Away From Negative People

Avoid people who, rather than encourage you to achieve your goals, laugh at them and invalidate your feelings. Avoid people who cause you pain intentionally and unintentionally.

Activity Six - Stop smoking or consuming hard drugs.

Activity Seven - Go to a park with friends and family.

Week Thirty-Five: Encouraging Words For Sick People

Visit a sick person this week and offer encouraging words to them.

Some encouraging words are:

"I hope you get better soon."

"It's a healing process. Don't rush things."

"Looking forward to seeing you back at work when you're better."

"You're in my thoughts every day as you recover from your illness."

"I love you and think of you all the time."

"I realize just how much I need you. So be strong for me!"

"You've been so brave handling this. You're my hero."

Week Thirty-Six: Dealing With Negative Feelings: Jealousy

Activity One – Find The Source

Think about your jealousy and the reason for it. You ought to have an idea of what the source is. When you do, please write it down.

Activity Two – Talk About Your Feelings

If your partner is doing something to make you feel jealous, you should talk about it with them, or you could talk about the source of your jealousy with someone you trust.

Activity Three – Turn The Negative Into Positive

Rather than let jealousy get the best of you. Decide to do positive things with it. If you're jealous of your best friend's new car, turn that jealousy into a passion and work towards getting a car for yourself too.

Activity Four – Look At Things From Another Perspective

What if there's no justification for you to be jealous. You're probably jealous of someone's fortune, but did you stop to wonder if they're unhappy with it?

Activity Five – Gratitude

Today, I need you to flashback to all you learned about gratitude during week seven's activities. Practice them today.

Activity Six – Take A Break

If you're working on overcoming something that triggers your jealousy, I suggest you take a break from it and things related to it. Also, walk away if you can.

Activity Seven – Always Take A Deep Breath

Feeling overwhelmed with thoughts of jealousy, take a deep breath and release. Repeat this process to calm your mind.

Week Thirty-Seven: Dealing With Negative Feelings: Anger

Activity One – Take Your Time To Think

When you're upset, you can say terrible things that people may never forget, so take your time to think thoroughly before speaking when provoked.

Activity Two – Express Your Anger Calmly

Try to calm yourself before expressing yourself. You could take a few breaths in, count from one to ten, walk away from the trigger. Just call yourself.

Activity Three – Exercise

If you're on the verge of getting angry, it's okay to take a walk or run.

Activity Four – Declare Positive Affirmations

"I can feel myself getting angry, but I choose to stay in control."

"I will remember to pause, stop and think before carrying out any action."

"I will not allow myself to perform an action I will regret."

Activity Five – Express Humor

Try listening to a joke when you're angry or even force yourself to laugh.

Activity Six – Let Go Of Grudges

Rather than piling up so much grudge in your heart, talk to the people who offended you about what they did.

Activity Seven – Seek Help

If you have an extreme anger issue, it's best to seek professional help.

Week Thirty-Eight: Dealing With Negative Feelings: Guilt

Activity One – Name Your Guilt

For example, *"I cheated on someone, and I feel terrible about it."*

"I feel bad that I yelled at a stranger who didn't deserve it."

Activity Two – Write Out The Roots Of It

Guilt could stem from things you've done, haven't done, or guilt-tripping from someone.

Activity Three – Apologize

Yes, say one of the magic words and tell the person you're sorry without making excuses.

Activity Four – Make Amends

It could be that your apology isn't enough at times, so go the extra mile to show that you're genuinely sorry. Make amends.

Activity Five – Learn

It could also be that whatever you did or whatever happened cannot be amended, so all you can choose to do is to learn from the past.

Activity Six – Gratitude

Oh yes, we're here again. Tell people you're thankful.

Activity Seven – Forgive Yourself

One of the things prolonging that guilt you always feel is guilt. Please, my dear black woman, forgive yourself.

Week Thirty-Nine: Dealing With Negative Feelings: Fear

Activity One - Take a deep breath in.

Activity Two – Learn about your fear

It might turn out that what you're afraid of really isn't anything to fear.

Activity Three – Stop Imagining Negative Things

Rather than expanding your fear by imagining the negative, use your imagination positively. Imagine happy places.

Activity Four - Engage in frequent meditations.

Activity Five – Be In Nature More Often

When you can't get the chance to talk to a therapist or friend about your fear, you could have some alone time in nature.

Activity Six - Use Your Fear To Your Advantage

Activity Seven – Make Goals

Write out five goals to achieve concerning your fear. For example, "I will address the crowd that I've feared all my life."

Week Forty: Dealing With Negative Feelings: Depression

Activity One – Don't Wallow Too Long

One of the reasons people fall into depression is wallowing too much in their sorrow. Feel that sadness but don't let it engulf you.

Activity Two – Embrace Hope

If what's currently happening is the cause of your depression, accept that tomorrow is unknown and be hopeful about it.

Activity Three – Stop Overgeneralizing

Stop thinking about all the wrong things in your life every time you forget that there have been some good times.

Activity Four – Drop That Weapon

There might be a voice that urges you to self-inflict. Do the exact opposite, drop that weapon.

Activity Five – Take A Break

Take a break from things stressing you out and adding to your depression.

Activity Six – Distract Yourself

Whenever you have depressive thoughts, take a walk, listen to music or chit-chat with a friend. Do things to distract you.

Activity Seven - Find a hobby you love doing.

Week Forty-One: Starting A Friendship

Activity One – Join A Group

Find a group with similar interests as yours and meet with them regularly.

Activity Two – Talk To Them

If you're interested in being friends with someone, you can start talking to them.

Activity Three – Accept Invitations

If you're invited by someone to hang out with them or a group of friends, it's okay to accept as long as you feel comfortable around them.

Activity Four – Smile Often

Activity Five – Talk About Yourself

If you're going to be friends with someone, they will have to know you, so you will feel okay talking about yourself with them. Also, ask them about themselves.

Activity Six – Carry Out Favors

The favors may seem little to you. It could be preparing their favorite meal, calling to ask how they are, etc. Show that you care.

Activity Seven – Don't Fake It.

It would be best if you didn't fake who you aren't to be friends with someone.

Week Forty-Two: Sustaining Friendships

Activity One - Call a friend you haven't heard from in a while.

Activity Two - Get a gift for each of your family members.

Activity Three - Get a gift for your friend.

Activity Four - Think of three friends that mean the world to you and write out five things you like about them.

Activity Five - Be honest with your friends.

If there's anyone you've lied to in the past, let them in on today's truth.

Activity Six – Encourage them.

If any of your friends are going through a lot now, send an encouraging message and let them know you care.

Activity Seven – Visitations

Most friendships grow stronger through communication and meetings. Call your friends and also try to visit the ones you can. You can also invite them to spend time with you.

Week Forty-Three: Getting Into A Relationship

Activity One – Be Clear About Your Intentions

Don't just get into relationships with people because of what you feel. Be certain of what you want with them and let them know. Know what they want too.

Activity Two – Have Self-Respect

Have respect for yourself and love yourself first. That way, you can respect and love someone else and know when someone is being unserious with you.

Activity Three – Move On

Write out things you need to move on from and work towards them before entering a relationship.

Activity Four – Avoid Peer Pressure

Don't enter a relationship because you're being pressured to. Be certain it's what you want.

Activity Five – Accept Your Partner

You shouldn't go into a relationship hoping that your partner will change a certain behavior. Either you accept their flaws and all or let them be.

Activity Six – Communicate

When you think about them, place a call and let them know they crossed your mind. Keep it moderate, though.

Activity Seven – Hang Out

Go to places with them and, observe how they react to things, note what they like and don't like. See if you feel at peace with them or not.

Week Forty-Four: Sustaining Your Relationship

Activity One – Continue The Communication

Don't relax because you're now dating or married to your partner. Still talk to them as much as you used to. Also, talk about things that matter to you both.

Activity Two – Be Dependable

Be someone your partner would always want to run to when they're troubled. Be someone they feel safe with.

Activity Three – Treat Yourself

Take out today to treat yourself specially. You can even ask your partner to take you on a treat.

Activity Four – Give Your Partner A Treat

Today is for your partner. Take them on a special treat and watch them smile throughout the day.

Activity Five – Say The Magic Words

"I'm sorry."

"Please."

"Thank you."

"You're welcome."

Activity Six – Spend Time With Your Partner

Create time out of your busy schedule to be with them. You could stay at home and watch a movie or play games or even go to a restaurant or their favorite place with them.

Activity Seven – Don't Be So Uptight.

Nobody wants to be around people who are always uptight and never find humor in anything. Do funny things, laugh with your partner and be happy.

Week Forty-Five: Understanding Sex and Sexual Intercourse

Activity One – Learn The Meaning

Write out the meaning of sex in your journal. Here's one meaning of sex from the Oxford Dictionary: a "sexual activity, including specifically sexual intercourse." You can research other definitions.

Activity Two – Know The types Of Sex

There are different kinds of sex. Vaginal, oral, anal sex, etc. Know about them.

Activity Three – Libido

What is libido?

How is it affected?

What affects it?

Activity Four – Learn About Consent

Consent is a very important keyword associated with sex. Learn about what it is and why it's important.

Activity Five – Use A Condom

Know about the type of protection to use when having sex to avoid STIs.

Activity Six – Learn About STIs

Know the full meaning of STIs. What they are, how they're transmitted, the stigma that follows, and everything about the topic.

Activity Seven – Know Your Partner's Sexual Choices

Learn about how your partner would rather have sex, which they would have sex with, do they have a fetish, etc.

Week Forty-Six: Preparing For Sex

Activity One – Give Hints

Let your partner know that you'd want to have sex before having sex, to avoid being unprepared.

Activity Two – Use Condoms

To avoid the transmission of STIs, always have a condom with you.

Activity Three – Lubricant Is Essential

Keep a lubricant next to your bed for easy reach while having sex.

Activity Four – Relax

You shouldn't have sex if you don't feel like it or feel tensed up. Try to relax first.

Activity Five – Slow And Steady

Starting slow will place you completely in the mood for sex and allow for easy penetration. Let your partner know that there's no need to rush.

Activity Six – Communicate Your Needs

If there's something you need before or while having sex, let your partner know. Always communicate if you need them to go faster or slower or stop completely.

Activity Seven – Spend Time With Your Partner

You do not necessarily have to talk always. Just snuggling up next to your partner and cuddling is needed sometimes.

Week Forty-Seven: Spicing Up Your Sex Life With Your Partner

Activity One – Keep your clothes on

Try something new. Rather than taking off your clothes completely, you could take off a few pieces and leave some. It can make you appear sexier to your partner.

Activity Two – Use Lubricant!

Using a flavored lubricant would make your partner want to go down completely on you for a very long time. It's great for sex.

Activity Three – Switch Locations.

Don't be boring. Try out different places for sex.

Activity Four - Try new positions with your partner.

It could be a wheelbarrow, 69, The leapfrog, etc.

Activity Five – Masturbate

Understand your body and know what makes you orgasm. That way, you can guide your partner.

Activity Six - Using a vibrator isn't a bad idea. Buy a premium one for better sex.

Activity Seven – Write Out Your Fantasies

Try to be creative and think about ways you'd like to have sex. Show your partner and agree on what to do together. Overall, have fun.

Week Forty-Eight: Voicing Out Affirmations 3

Activity One – Affirmations For Sexual Confidence

"I embrace my sexuality and accept who I am."

"I am breathtaking."

"I deserve the gift of sexual pleasure."

Activity Two – Affirmations For Body Positivity

"I won't starve myself in a bid to get a slimmer body."

"I love every part of my body and think they're awesome."

"Comparing myself to others is a sign of low-self esteem. I won't cultivate that habit."

Activity Three – Affirmations For Beauty

"I love my eyes. They're captivating."

"I am incredibly sexy."

"I love my black skin because it's beautiful."

Activity Four – Affirmations For A Great Sex Life

"My body makes my partner go wild whenever he sees me."

"My body deserves all the touches, caresses and pleasure it gets."

"Sex is a sacred activity that the partner I choose and I have decided to engage in."

Activity Five – Affirmations For Sex Drive

"I am charged with sexual energy."

"I accept sex as a part of my life."

"None of my sexual experiences will be bland."

Activity Six – Affirmations For Seduction

"I am tuned in to male/female signals."

"I am confident with my partner."

"My seduction skills are becoming powerful."

Activity Seven – Affirmations For Dating

"I am worthy of love and respect that anyone gives."

"I will find the perfect one who would love and cherish me."

"I am capable of giving love to people."

Week Forty-Nine: Embracing Your Sexuality

Activity One – Do What Makes You Happy

Rather than worry about what people would say about your sexuality, why not do what makes you happy, what you care about? Dance in a weird way, dress crazily, whatever makes you happy.

Activity Two – Embrace Your Body

If you're putting on clothes to avoid seeing your body, then you have to stop. Observe and admire yourself in the mirror and smile at how beautiful you are.

Activity Three – Fall In Love With Yourself

For you to love someone, you have to love yourself first. Remember your spiritual journey.

Activity Four – Stop Following The Media

The media says to do this, and you do it even to your unhappiness. That's a really bad path to follow. Stop listening to people who have barely lived their life telling you how to live yours.

Activity Five – Sex Positivity

Listen to podcasts like Why Are People Into That, read Lisa Taddeo's Three Women. Follow books that encourage sex-positivity.

Activity Six – You Should Feel Great

Sexuality and sex should make you feel great and not less of yourself. So if you feel otherwise after having sex with your partner, it's a sign that's not it.

Activity Seven – Accept Your Sexuality

Understand that God isn't ashamed of your sexuality because he made you who you are. So if he's okay with it, why shouldn't you be?

Week Fifty: Preparing For A Vacation

I planned a vacation for you for weeks fifty-one to fifty-two, which is two weeks. I don't know what time is suitable for you so that you can adjust it. But my dear black woman, try as much as you can to go on a vacation before the year runs out. Take a rest and feel refreshed.

Activity One – Save Up

Start by planning your budget and saving up for your vacation.

Activity Two – Ask Questions

Wherever you have in mind to travel to, it's best to do your research on it, foods you could try, places you could go, etc.

Activity Three – Use A Checklist

As you pack, you mustn't overpack and also not under-pack. So have a checklist which you would work with to ensure you pack all you need.

Activity Four – Check The Weather

Some countries might have unfavorable weather by the time you wish to travel. Do your best to check the weather and plan according to it.

Activity Five - Pay off any outstanding bills before you leave.

Rather than piling up your bills while away, it's best to pay them off. You're going on a vacation to refresh your body and mind; it wouldn't be nice to return refreshed only to be cramped up with bills to pay.

Activity Six – Notify Your Bank

It would help if you always remembered to call your bank and inform them of your travel days and where you're traveling to ensure your credit card remains active in the country you intend to visit.

Activity Seven – Leave Your Home In Shape

Unplug electronics, turn off the lights, turn off the tap, etc. Make sure your home is in order before traveling.

Week Fifty-One – Week Fifty-Two: Vacation Week!

Conclusion

My dear black woman, I had an exhilarating experience writing this book for you. I hope you had a fun time reading through it, too. I hope you learnt, and I hope all that you learned stays with you for a very long time.

Every day society tries to shun black women by telling them what their spirituality and sexuality should be and what they shouldn't be. But the truth remains that no one can define your spirituality for you. Same as your sexuality. These are two important things that you define and experience by yourself.

This book mirrors my journey as a black woman who chooses not to let the world affect her spiritual and sexual self. Every word is me telling my truth and living it. It took a long time to get this far.

I hope this book helps you too. I hope you become your most audacious, daring, spiritual, and adventurous self. You are so dearly and deeply loved.

Thank You

You could have picked from dozens of other books, but you picked our book

Powerful Hypnotic Affirmations and Spiritual Self-Care for Black Women

So, THANK YOU so much for getting this book and for making it all the way to the end.

Could you please consider posting a review on Amazon or Audible if you picked the audio version as well?

Posting a review is the best and easiest way to support the work of independent authors like us.

Your feedback will help us to keep writing the kind of books that will help you get the results you want.

It can be something short and simple ☺

www.ingramcontent.com/pod-product-compliance
Lightning Source LLC
Chambersburg PA
CBHW072043110526
44590CB00018B/3020